Color Atlas of

E.N.T.
Diagnosis

Third edition

T. R. Bull
FRCS
Consultant Surgeon
Royal National Throat Nose and Ear Hospital, London
Senior Lecturer to the Institute of Laryngology & Otology
Consultant Surgeon, Charing Cross Hospital, London
Consultant Surgeon, King Edward VII Hospital for
Officers, London

D1392755

M Mosby-Wolfe

London Baltimore Bogotá Boston Buenos Aires Caracas Carlsbad, CA Chicago Madrid Mexico City Milan Naples, FL New York Philadelphia St. Louis Sydney Tokyo Toronto Wiesbaden

Project Manager:	Jane Hurd-Cosgrave
Developmental Editor:	Lucy Hamillton
Layout Artist:	Jane Hurd-Cosgrave
Cover Design:	Ian Spick
Illustration:	Lynda Payne
Production:	Mike Heath
Index:	Anita Reid
Publisher:	Geoff Greenwood

CONTENTS

PREFACE

It is eight years since the publication of the previous edition of *Colour Atlas of ENT Diagnosis*. In this time, improvements in radiological investigation and surgical techniques have been developed for many ear and sinus conditions, and this, along with the need for a better presentation, calls for an updated edition.

CT scanning and magnetic resonance imaging have become routine for help in diagnosis of many head and neck, ear and sinus pathologies. Fibreoptic instruments for examination of the upper respiratory tract are standard, and endoscopic sinus techniques have brought modern keyhole surgery to the nose and added precision, particularly to operations of the ethmoid sinus.

The basic format of this atlas, however, remains unaltered. The aim is to give a pictorial survey of the speciality with a succinct text to be of practical help in diagnosis. It is not intended to be an illustrated textbook, and reference to larger texts is needed for a more thorough knowledge of the conditions illustrated. This revised atlas will, I hope, continue to stimulate the interest of medical students in this speciality, and also give useful, practical information to ENT trainees and to those in general practice and casualty, where ENT conditions so commonly present. It also contains information which hopefully will be of relevance and help to those in allied specialties.

T. R. Bull

ACKNOWLEDGEMENTS

Most of the photographs in this book were taken by myself, but I am grateful for the expertise of the Photographic Department of the Royal National Throat Nose & Ear Hospital for many of the better illustrations. My thanks also to my colleagues, who kindly contributed the following illustrations: Professor Tony Wright, 156, 170; Mr David Howard, 184; Miss Valerie Lund, 298, 299; Mr David Proops, 83; Dr Van Hasselt, 334; Professor Weerda, 80. 82; Dr Glyn Lloyd, 203; Dr Pedro Claros, 452; Mr Tony Cheesman, 444; Dr A. H. Davis, 121; Mr John Evans, 428; Mr Charles Smith, 164; Dr J. Brennand, 205; Dr E. Scadding, 54, 55. Illustration no. 409 has been reprinted with permission from Dr Charles F. Farthing, *Color Atlas of AIDS and HIV Disease, 2nd Edn.*, 1988, Mosby–Wolfe, London.

The book has been perused by Mr Martin Bailey, a colleague at the Royal National Throat Nose and Ear Hospital, whom I would like to thank him for his advice on the text and content. I would also like to thank Mrs. Jean Roussel for advice on the audiometry section.

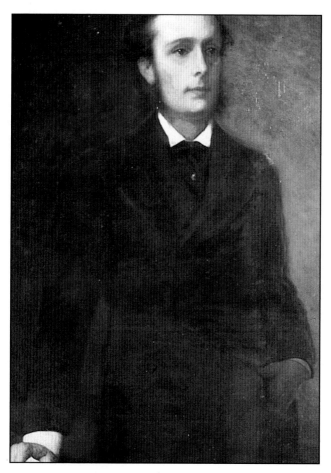

Sir Morrell MacKenzie

This painting shows the austere Scottish physician and surgeon who founded Ear, Nose and Throat as a speciality and wrote the first standard textbook on Rhinology and Laryngology. Sir Morrell MacKenzie also founded one of the first hospitals for Nose and Throat diseases in London in 1863 (today the Royal National Throat Nose and Ear Hospital). The most common condition he treated in this hospital was laryngeal tuberculosis, at that time invariably fatal, but today rare and curable.

Chapter 1

ENT Examination

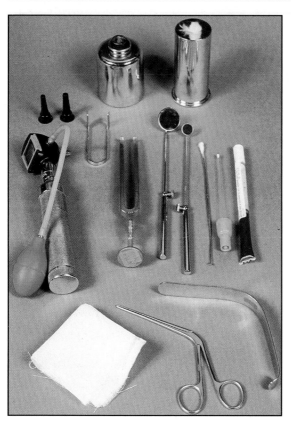

1 The instruments needed for an ENT examination: The *laryngeal and post-nasal mirrors* require warming to avoid misting, and hot water or a spirit lamp is necessary. An angled *tongue depressor* or wooden spatula is needed for examining the oropharynx and post-nasal space. *Angled forceps* are used for dressing the nose or ear. A *tuning fork* is essential for the diagnosis of conductive or sensori-neural (perceptive) hearing loss. A C1 or C2 (256 or 512 cps) is needed. The very large tuning forks used to test vibration sense are unsatisfactory, and may give a false Rinne test. A *Jobson–Horne probe* is widely used in ENT departments. A loop on one end is for removing wax (and foreign bodies) from the ear or nose. Cotton wool attached to the other end is used for cleaning the ear. An *auriscope*, *nasal* and *aural specula* complete the basic instruments.

A *sterile swab* and *media* are necessary for throat, nasal or ear specimens to be taken for culture and sensitivity. A 'narrow' swab holder as shown here is extremely useful for aural specimens, as the more common swab is too wide and can be traumatic for the deep meatus and middle ear.

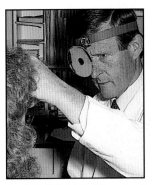 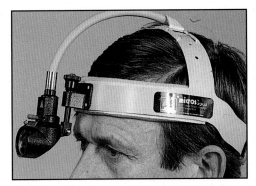

2, 3 Lighting. The *head mirror* (**2, left**) gives effective lighting for examining the upper respiratory tract and ear, and leaves both hands free for using instruments. Initially, the technique of using a head mirror is not easy, and some may prefer a *fibreoptic* or *electric headlight* (**3, right**).

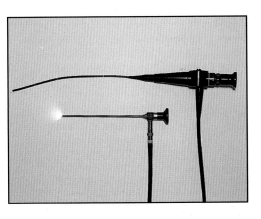

4 Rigid and flexible fibreoptic endoscopes. These are important additional examination instruments. The flexible endoscope is of value to see the laryngeal region (see **68**) in those with a marked gag reflux in whom indirect laryngoscopy (see **67**) with a mirror is difficult. The rigid endoscope is important in examination of the nasal cavities.

EXAMINATION OF THE EAR

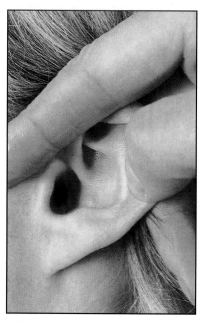 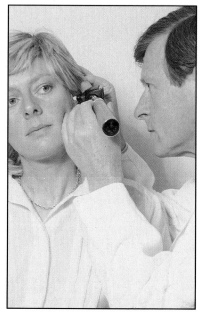

5 Retracting the pinna. The meatus is tortuous. Therefore, to see the drum the pinna is retracted backwards and outwards, and the index finger may be used to hold the tragus forward.

6 The auriscope. This is best held like a pen. In this way, the examiner's little finger can rest on the patient's cheek; if the patient's head moves, the position of the ear speculum is maintained in the meatus.

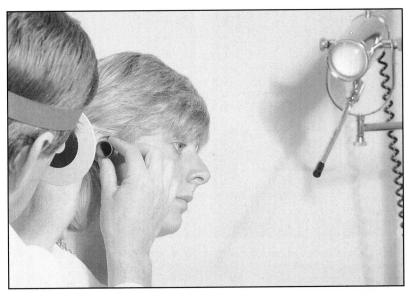

7 Head mirror and speculum. These are used for the initial examination of the meatus and drum.

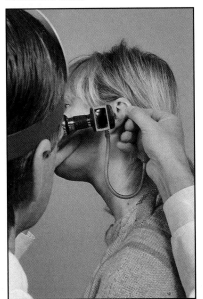

8 A pneumatic otoscope. A hand-held air-filled bulb attached to the auriscope enables air to be gently inflated against the drum for demonstrating drum mobility. Reduced mobility is conspicuous, and is diagnostic of middle-ear fluid. Reduced mobility is also seen with tympano-sclerosis, or with a drum that may be of a normal appearance but in which there is malleus fixation.

The *fistula test* may be made with the pneumatic otoscope. Pressure change by pressing on the bulb will cause dizziness with nystagmus (*positive fistula sign*) in those with erosion of the labyrinth by cholesteatoma (see **157**) or with a perilymph fistula.

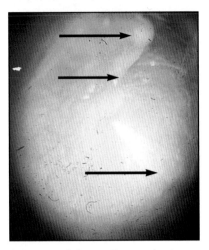

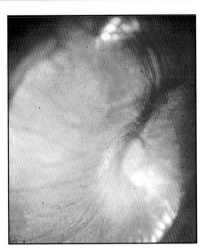

9 A normal drum. The main land-marks seen on the pars tensa of a normal drum are the lateral process *(top arrow)* and handle *(middle arrow)* of the malleus, and the light reflex *(lower arrow)*. The drum superior to the short process is the pars flaccida or attic part of the drum. A normal drum is grey, and varies in vascularity and translucency.

10 A more vascular drum. This has vessels extending down the handle of the malleus to the umbo.

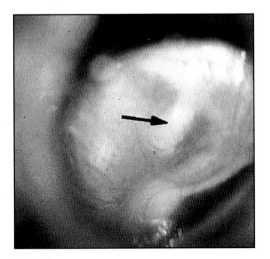

11 The incus *(arrow)* may show as a shadow through a thin drum, as may the round window and opening of the Eustachian tube, although this is less common.

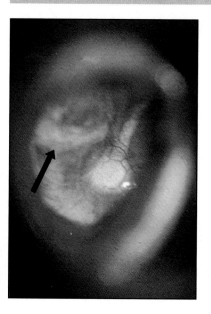

12 The chorda tympani nerve is the nerve giving taste to the anterior two-thirds of the tongue (excluding the circumvallate papillae), and is also the secretomotor nerve to the submandibular and sublingual salivary glands.

The chorda tympani nerve usually lies behind the pars flaccida (*arrow*). It is not normally visible, but if the nerve is more inferior it shows through the drum.

If examination of the drum and meatus is normal in a patient complaining of earache, the pain is *referred*. **Referred ear pain** may be from nearby structures such as the temporo-mandibular joint, neck muscles or cervical spine. It may also be from the teeth, tongue, tonsils or larynx. The Vth, IXth and Xth cranial nerves which supply these sites have their respective tympanic and auricular branches supplying the ear. Earache also frequently precedes a Bell's palsy.

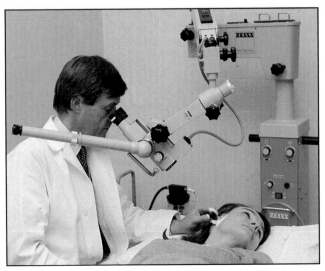

13 Microscope examination of the drum. Although most drums can be seen well and conditions diagnosed with the auriscope, the increased magnification that is obtainable with the operating microscope is sometimes necessary, and this apparatus is standard for a well-equipped out-patient department.

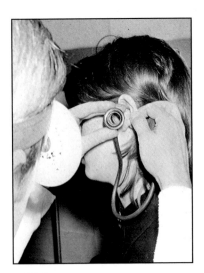

14 Siegle's speculum has been displaced by the pneumatic otoscope (see **8**), but Siegle's speculum with plain (not magnifying) glass is extremely useful to test drum mobility with the microscope.

HEARING LOSS

Most hearing loss is easy to diagnose as either a well-defined conductive or sensori-neural type. ('Mixed' hearing loss may occur, but this diagnosis is usually non-contributory, and the term is better avoided.)

Lesions to the left of the blue line (**15**, below) cause conductive hearing loss, and are frequently curable; hearing loss to the right of the blue line is due to a sensori-neural lesion, and is usually not so amenable to treatment.

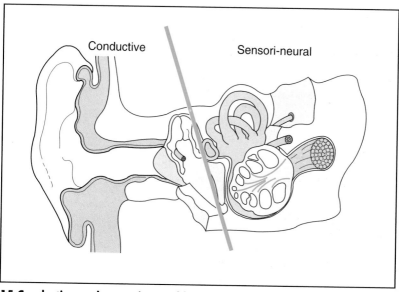

15 Conductive and sensori-neural hearing loss. Hearing loss is either conductive or sensori-neural in type; it is an essential basic step in diagnosis of hearing loss to distinguish between these two. Sensori-neural hearing loss is either due to a cochlear or retro-cochlear lesion.

Tests for conductive and sensori-neural hearing loss

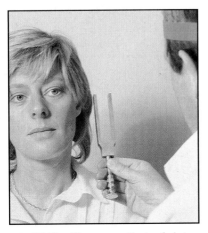 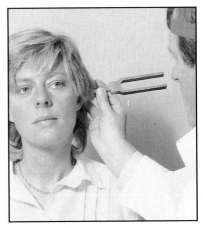

16, 17 The Rinne test. Tuning fork tests are essential preliminary tests for the diagnosis of hearing loss.

The Rinne and Weber tests enable the diagnosis of a conductive or sensori-neural hearing loss to be made. If the tuning fork is heard louder on the mastoid process than in front of the ear, the Rinne is negative, and the hearing loss conductive. If the tuning fork is heard better in front of the ear, the Rinne is positive, and the hearing is either normal or there is sensori-neural hearing loss.

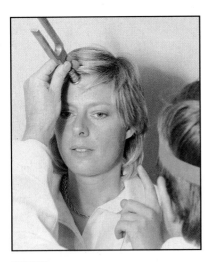

18 The Weber test. The tuning fork, when held in the mid-line on the forehead, is heard in the ear with the conductive hearing loss. This test is very sensitive, and if the meatus is occluded with the finger, the tuning fork will be heard in that ear. A conductive loss of as little as five decibels will result in the Weber being referred to that ear.

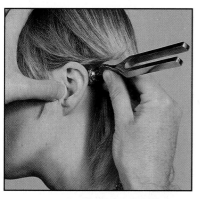

19 The occlusion test (Bing). This is also helpful. The tuning fork is held on the mastoid process and the tragus lightly pushed to occlude the meatus. The tuning fork is heard louder. In conductive hearing loss, even of a slight degree, there is no change when the meatus is occluded. The Rinne test does not become negative until there is a marked degree of conductive loss (about a 20-decibel air–bone gap). It is therefore possible to have a slight conductive hearing loss with a positive Rinne. The more sensitive occlusion test will help in the diagnosis.

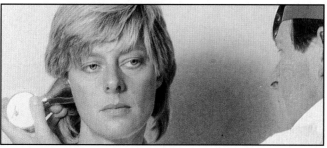

20 Barany box. This is used to confirm total hearing loss. It is placed on the good ear, and produces a noise totally masking this ear. The patient will be unable to repeat words clearly spoken into the deaf ear.

Total hearing loss in one ear

Total hearing loss in one ear is frequently wrongly diagnosed as a conductive hearing loss. The Rinne is negative because the tuning fork, although not heard in front of the ear, is heard by the better ear when placed on the mastoid process of the deaf ear, with the sound being transmitted by the bone (*false-negative Rinne*). The Weber test gives the clue that the Rinne is false, as the sound will not lateralise to the deaf ear.

Total hearing loss in one ear may be congenital or the result of a skull fracture. Meningitis is also a cause, but **mumps** is probably the commonest cause.

An acoustic neuroma presents with a unilateral sensori-neural loss, which may become total. If this hearing loss is associated with a canal paresis on the caloric test and an enlarged internal auditory meatus on x-ray, an acoustic tumour is probable. These are basic preliminary tests in the diagnosis of acoustic neuroma.

Hearing aids

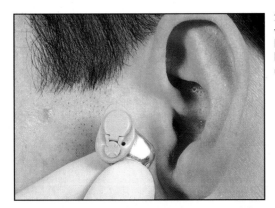

21 Hearing aids. Aids worn to **both** ears may be helpful. The **better** ear may be preferred if only one aid is used.

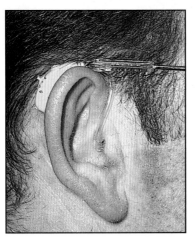 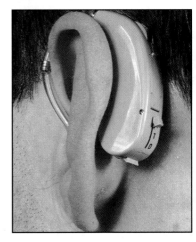

22, 23 Hearing aids. Conductive hearing loss that is not amenable to surgical treatment responds well to conventional hearing aids, as may sensori-neural hearing loss with a 'flat' tracing, in which the hearing loss is equal at most frequencies.

Most commonly, however, sensori-neural hearing loss affects the high tones, with relatively good hearing at the low frequencies. There are still difficulties to overcome in designing a hearing aid that can provide good speech discrimination for this type of hearing loss. Aids containing a microphone, amplifier, battery and earphone can be fitted either behind the ear, to spectacles or, in certain cases, as an in-the-ear aid.

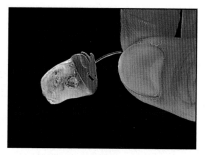
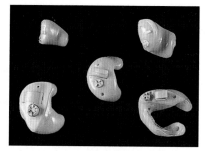

24, 25 Modern hearing aids are so small that they may be fitted completely within the ear canal, either adjacent to the tympanic membrane or 'semi-deep'. These aids are for mild-to-moderate hearing loss. With severe hearing loss, a behind-the-ear aid is needed, and a body-worn aid is used for profound hearing loss and for those lacking the dexterity to manipulate a small aid.

Patience and advice are needed to adapt to the use of a hearing aid, and in this and other forms of hearing loss management, **_hearing therapists_** have an important role.

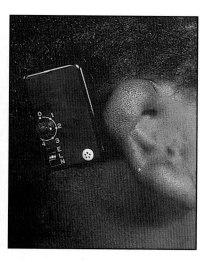

26 Bone-anchored hearing aid. The aid clips onto osseo-integrated titanium screws fixed to the mastoid bone. It is an efficient sound conductor for those with congenital absence or deformity of the ear canal and pinna, in whom a conventional hearing aid cannot be fitted.

With ear discharge not controlled medically or surgically, the fitting of a conventional aid for conductive hearing loss is also not practical, and bone-anchored aids may be used.

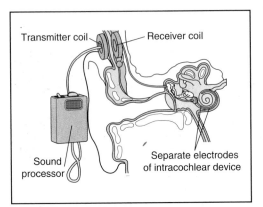

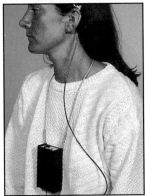

27, 28 Implants for total hearing loss. Total or profound hearing loss involving both ears has stimulated innovative surgery to develop an electronic ***cochlear implant***. At present, techniques achieve an appreciation of sound for those who were previously totally deaf. A cochlear implant may help those with total or profound hearing loss, for which the most powerful aid is ineffective (e.g. deafness due to meningitis, head injury or ototoxic drugs). **27** (left) shows a multichannel intracochlear implant in position.

An ear-level microphone is fitted like a hearing aid. Sound is converted to electric signals by a body-worn speech processor (**28**, right) and transmitted to electrodes inserted surgically into the cochlea. With a good result, hearing is such that a telephone may be used.

Investigation of hearing loss: radiology

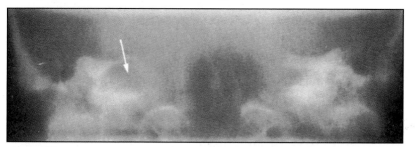

29 Acoustic neuroma. A unilateral sensori-neural hearing loss may be caused by an acoustic neuroma. In the past, when the hearing loss was not investigated, acoustic neuromas were diagnosed late when they were large with other more obvious symptoms and signs of a space-occupying intracranial lesion. There is now a marked awareness that sensori-neural loss, particularly if unilateral and even if minimal, requires investigation to exclude acoustic neuroma.

Polytomogram x-rays of the internal auditory meatus (associated with an absent or im-paired caloric response—see **43**) are helpful preliminary investigations in the diag-nosis of an acoustic neuroma. *Arrow* indicates the enlarged internal auditory meatus.

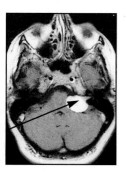
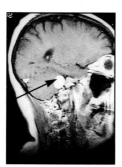

30, 31 CT and MRI scans. Two important x-ray innovations developed in Great Britain are the **CT** (computerised tomo-graphy) (**30**, left) and **MRI** (magnetic resonance imaging) (**31**, right) scans. These are very helpful in the diagnosis of acoustic neuroma *(arrows)*.

Magnetic resonance imaging is the single most important investigation for acoustic neuroma. Early diagnosis is important for a small neuroma (less than 1 cm in diameter); this can be removed with preservation of the facial nerve to which it is adjacent in the internal auditory meatus, and the hearing too may be preserved.

Neuromas arise from the nerve sheath (strictly termed 'schwannomas'), and may be dissected from the auditory nerve. The prognosis for larger neuromas is less good, with risk of permanent damage to the facial nerve and increased morbidity from intracranial surgery.

Investigation of hearing loss: audiometry

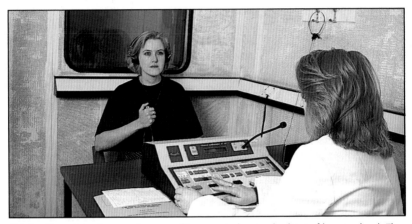

32 Audiometry. A *pure-tone audiogram* is the standard test of hearing level. The readings are recorded on a chart with intensity (0–100 dB) and frequency (usually 250–8000 cps). A normal tracing is between –10 dB and +10 dB at all frequencies. This test is accurate to about 10 dB only, as there are variables due to the patient's responses and the accuracy of both the audiometrician and the machine.

Hearing is tested in front of the ear (air conduction—recorded in black) and over the mastoid process (bone conduction—in red). A silent or sound-proof room is necessary for accurate pure-tone audiometry.

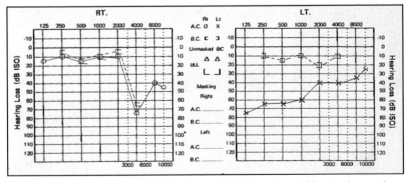

33 Audiograms. The one on the left shows a typical sensori-neural hearing loss; a sharp dip at 4000 cps, as on this chart, is typical of inner ear damage due to **noise trauma**.

A loss of high frequencies is commonly seen in hearing loss of old age (**presbycousis**). The audiogram on the right shows a conductive hearing loss with the sound heard better on the bone, typical of **otosclerosis** or **otitis media**.

Audiometry requires skill and training, particularly to test children. An audiogram is obtainable from most children by the age of 3–4 years. With unilateral hearing loss, noise is used to mask the better ear, so that this ear does not hear the sound transmission from the deaf ear and give a false reading. Hearing assessment under the age of 3 years, or in children who are unable to cooperate with audiometry, requires special skills and techniques.

The response of a baby or toddler to meaningful sounds, such as a spoon 'chinked' against a cup, gives an indication of hearing. ***Electrocochleography*** (ECoG) involves placing fine electrodes through the drum to pick up auditory nerve reaction potential in response to sound. This refined test gives a good hearing assessment for infants in whom a hearing loss is suspected. Anaesthesia is required for electrocochleography. This objective test of hearing acuity is also of help in the diagnosis of psychosomatic hearing loss or malingering. The ***auditory brain stem response*** (ABR), in which electroencephalogram recordings are made following auditory stimulus, is another useful audiometric test.

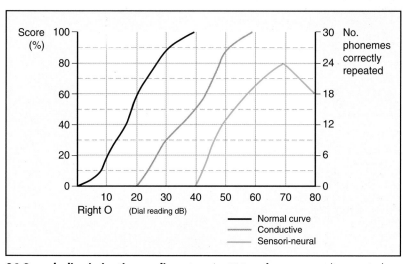

34 Speech discrimination audiometry. A criticism of pure-tone audiometry is that an assessment of the ability to hear pure-tone sounds may not reflect the ability to hear speech. A phonetically balanced list of words is used. The percentage of those correctly detected is used as the index to plot a speech discrimination chart. The ability to understand speech is obviously reduced with all hearing loss but particularly with sensori-neural loss in which the high tones are involved. An additional help in the diagnosis of acoustic neuromas may be poor speech discrimination, in excess of that expected from the level of the pure-tone audiogram.

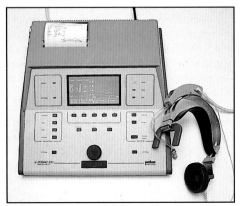

35 Impedance audiometry involves performing several measurements to obtain a wide range of information about the middle and inner ear.

A probe with a rubber tip and containing three small patent tubes is fitted into the meatus to make an airtight seal. One tube delivers the tone to the ear, a second tube is attached to a microphone to monitor the sound pressure level within the ear canal, and a third tube is attached to a manometer to vary the air pressure in the ear.

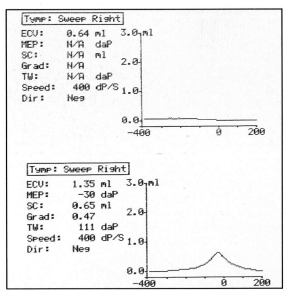

36 Impedance measurements are particularly helpful in the differential diagnosis of conductive and sensori-neural hearing losses, as they give information about middle-ear pressure, Eustachian tube function, middle-ear reflexes, and the level of a lower motor-neurone facial nerve palsy. Impedance testing is now widely used to confirm the presence of middle-ear fluid, and the 'flat' tracing is characteristic. A 'glue ear' may be diagnosed in babies and younger children using impedance measurements when the cooperation required for a pure-tone audiogram is not possible.

TESTS OF BALANCE

Vertigo is most commonly due to a disorder of the labyrinth. A sensation of unsteadiness may occur, however, with hypoglycaemia, orthostatic hypotension, hyperventilation and cerebral ischaemia. Tumours or multiple sclerosis involving the vestibular system also cause imbalance.

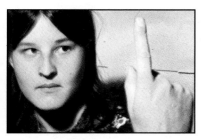

37 Observation for nystagmus is one of the clinical tests for abnormalities of balance. Nystagmus due to a labyrinth disorder is characterised by a slow and quick phase of eye movement in which the eye moves slowly away from the side of the involved labyrinth, then flicks rapidly back to that side; the nystagmus is said to be in the direction of the quick phase. The eye movement in nystagmus is fine.

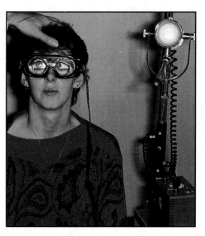

38 Frenzel glasses. Observation of nystagmus is facilitated by fitting the patient with glasses having magnifying lenses, such as Frenzel glasses.

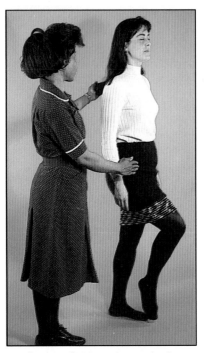 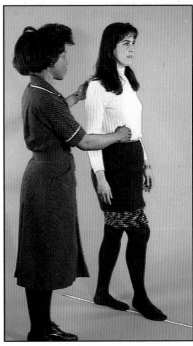

39 The Romberg test is another basic test of balance. This test, in which the patient is asked to stand still with feet together and eyes closed, is made more sensitive by asking the patient to mark time, when instability is obvious, indicating a significant balance disorder.

40 Tests to demonstrate abnormalities of gait. One of these is heel–toe walking along a straight line. A person with normal balance is stable without looking down at the feet.

Abnormalities in these preliminary clinical tests of balance will indicate the need for further investigation.

Vertigo due to a labyrinth disorder may occur with or without hearing loss.

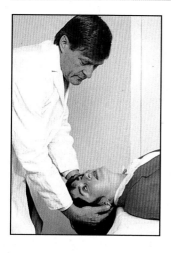

41 Positional vertigo.

Positional vertigo (the positional test)

Benign paroxysmal positional vertigo is a sudden and severe rotary vertigo, occurring when lying down in bed or upon looking upwards, when the head is placed backwards and to one side. There is no hearing loss, and it may follow a head injury. Although common, it is frequently not recognised, and unnecessary neurological investigation may be carried out.

The positional history is typical, and diagnosis is confirmed by a positive positional test. When the head is placed backwards and to one side, there is nystagmus which fatigues within several seconds, but recurs temporarily when the patient sits up.

This is a self-limiting condition, and advising the patient simply to avoid the position that triggers off the attack may suffice as treatment. Positional vertigo may also occur with space-occupying lesions involving the cerebellum and cerebello-pontine angle. Nystagmus may be induced with the positional test, but there is no latent period and the nystagmus does not fatigue.

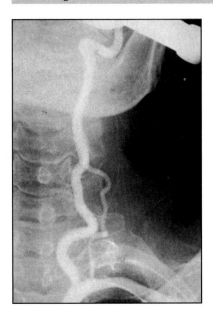

42 Vertebro-basilar ischaemia.
Vertigo with head movement, or transient sudden loss of consciousness ('drop' attacks), occur with temporary interruption of the blood supply to the labyrinth or cerebral cortex. This condition is seen in older patients with cervical osteoarthritis, and with evidence of hypertension and atherosclerosis. Movement of the irregular cervical spine temporarily occludes the tortuous atherosclerotic vertebral vessels which lead to the basilar and internal auditory arteries.

This **vertebral angiogram** shows the kinking of the vertebral artery.

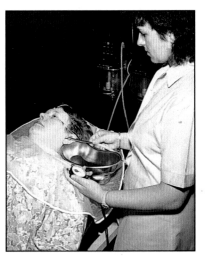

43 The caloric test. Irrigation of the external meatus with water 7° above and later 7° below body temperature sets up convection currents of the endolymph in the semicircular canals. This causes nystagmus, and the duration of the nystagmus gives an index of the activity of the labyrinth. The nystagmus can be directly observed or recorded electrically **(electronystagmography)**. This test is particularly valuable in the diagnosis of Ménière's disease and acoustic neuroma. A reduced or absent nystagmus is found (canal paresis).

Ménière's disease

Sudden severe rotary vertigo often with nausea and vomiting, a ***tinnitus*** increasing prior to the vertigo, and a ***sensori-neural hearing loss*** (cochlear type) form the triad of symptoms characteristic of ***Ménière's disease*** (**44**).

In this curious condition, there is an increase in the endolymph volume, but the cause is unknown. The disease has a reputation for being serious which is not justified. Although the vertigo may occasionally be severe and incapacitating, the symptoms are frequently mild, usually self-limiting and not progressive. It is never fatal, and medical treatment with labyrinthine sedatives, e.g. prochlorperazine, commonly controls the vertigo. Oral histamine-like drugs which aim to increase the blood flow to the inner ear (e.g. betahistine) may also be effective, but there is no proven specific medical therapy at present available for Ménière's.

Many innovative surgical procedures have been tried; none of them have proved to be totally successful, although decompression of the endolymphatic sac in an attempt to reduce the pressure in the scala media is the present favoured conservative surgery. Surgery to destroy the labyrinth is effective in controlling the vertigo, but an irreversible total hearing loss with accentuated tinnitus is one of the factors that make this treatment a last resort.

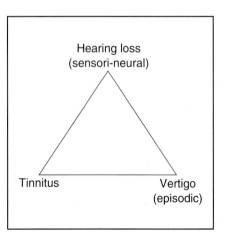

44 The triad of Ménière's disease.

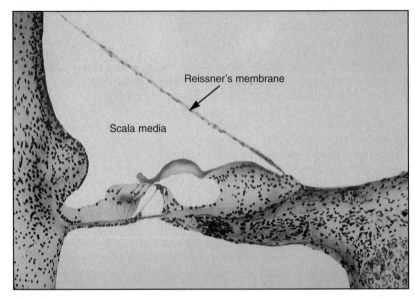

45 Normal ear.

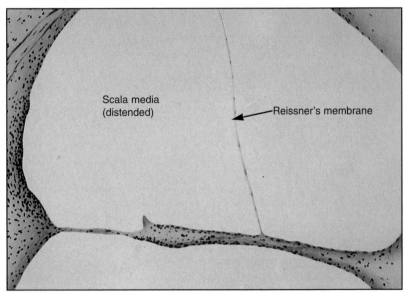

46 Ménière's disease.

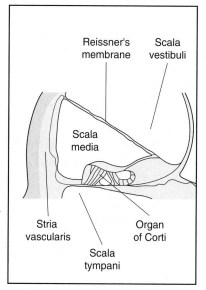

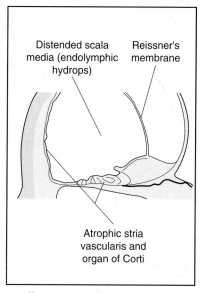

47 Illustration of normal ear.

48 Illustration of ear with Ménière's disease.

Tinnitus

Tinnitus is commonly associated with hearing loss, although it may rarely be troublesome with normal hearing. Tinnitus with conductive hearing loss is usually less distressing than tinnitus with sensori-neural hearing loss, as in the latter the tinnitus may cause serious psychiatric disturbance. The full physiology and pathology of tinnitus remains unknown, and there is no entirely effective treatment. Explanation and reassurance are helpful in the patient's acceptance of tinnitus (patients frequently associate it with serious intracranial disease), and the use of a tranquillizer may be necessary.

Tinnitus-maskers, in which a hearing aid–like device feeds a noise that has been matched with the tinnitus into the ear, may mask the tinnitus to a greater or lesser degree and be effective as a treatment. Surgical treatment of tinnitus with section of the acoustic nerve or destruction of the inner ear has been tried and is unsatisfactory.

EXAMINATION OF THE NOSE

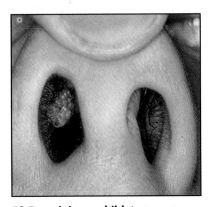

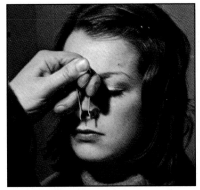

49 Examining a child. Instruments are best avoided in children; a good anterior view of the nose can be obtained simply by pressing on the tip of the nose. In this case, a clear view is obtained of a pedunculated papilloma of the nasal vestibule.

50 Speculum examination shows the nasal vestibule, the septum anteriorly (particularly Little's area—see **310**), and the inferior and middle turbinates anteriorly. There are several different types of nasal speculum used throughout the world. (The one demonstrated here is the Thudicum speculum.)

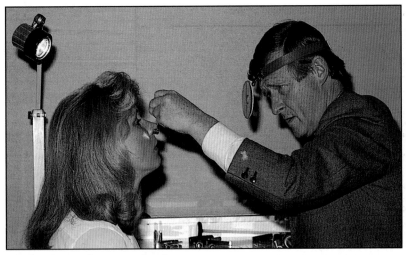

51 Nasal speculum examination.

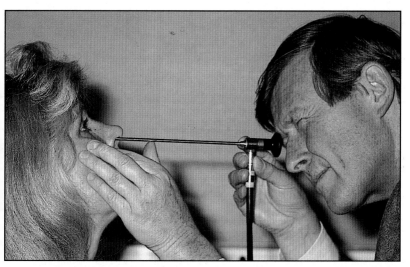

52 A nasal endoscope is necessary for a thorough examination of the nasal cavities, the mucosa having been sprayed with surface anaesthetic.

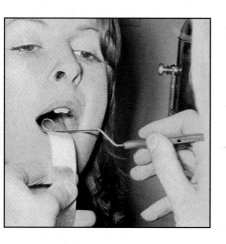

53 Mirror examination of the post-nasal space. This is not easy, particularly in children. With a patient who gags easily, or whose soft palate is close to the posterior wall of the oropharynx, a view may be impossible.

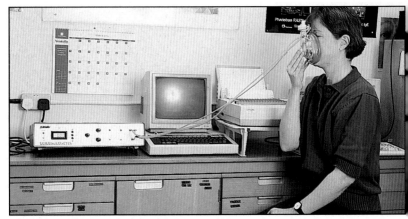

54 Rhinomanometry techniques give a quantitative measurement of nasal airway. Many methods have been employed, but the anterior active method has gained most acceptance. The pressure is measured through one nostril, while the flow is measured through the opposite side using a face mask and pneumotach.

Rhinomanometry has yet to become of sufficient clinical value to be of routine use in the assessment of nasal obstruction, as the threshold of nasal obstruction or 'congestion' of which the patient complains correlates poorly with air pressure measurements.

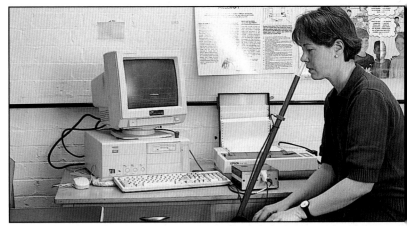

55 Acoustic rhinomanometry. Noise introduced into the nasal vestibule is reflected from the interior of the nose. With a widely patent nasal airway, the reflection of sound is delayed and less intense than with nasal obstruction. Hence, a graph of normality can be made, and acoustic rhinometry is one recent objective measurement for nasal airway.

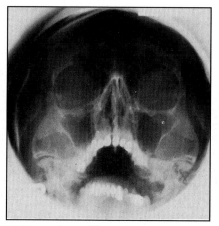

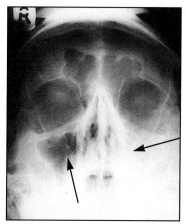

57

56 Normal maxillary sinus x-ray.

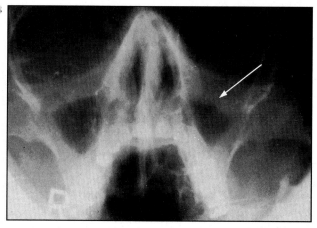

56–58 X-rays showing maxillary sinuses. An x-ray will show opacity (**57**, *right arrow*) suggesting infection or polyposis, or opacity with bone destruction suggestive of a neoplasm. The polypoid swelling (shown here in the floor of the right antrum (**57**, *right arrow*), or thickening of the antral mucosa (**58**, *arrow*) are frequent chance findings, and in the absence of symptoms or other signs are probably not significant. A straight anterior-posterior x-ray will show the ethmoid and frontal sinuses, and a lateral and base of skull view the sphenoid sinus.

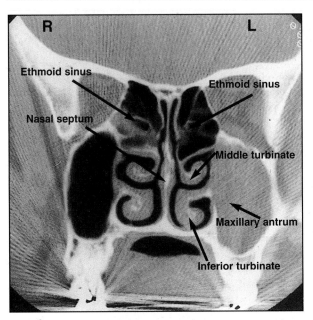

R   L

Ethmoid sinus

Ethmoid sinus

Nasal septum

Middle turbinate

Maxillary antrum

Inferior turbinate

59 A CT scan of the sinuses gives precise detail, particularly of the ethmoids, which are not well seen on the plain x-ray. The CT scan is important prior to sinus surgery. The left maxillary antrum is seen to be opaque on this x-ray from infection, but the left ethmoids are clear. Some minimal mucosal thickening (which would not be detected on plain x-rays) is seen in the right ethmoid sinus.

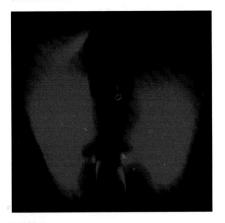

60 Transillumination. A bright light held inside the mouth in a dark room is an investigation rarely used. A dull antrum is, however, an additional sign in the diagnosis of maxillary sinus disease. Transillumination is useful to assess whether a sinusitis is settling. Dental cysts involving the antrum transilluminate brightly.

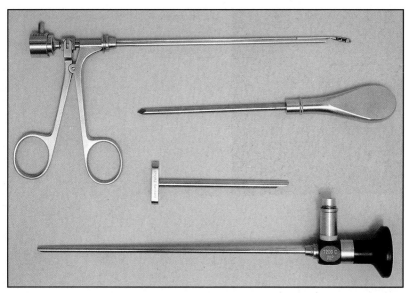

61 Sinus endoscopy (antroscopy). A narrow endoscope inserted into the maxillary antrum, either through the thin bony wall of the canine fossa intra-orally or via the inferior meatus of the nasal fossa under the inferior turbinate, gives a good view of the interior of the maxillary sinus, and is helpful in diagnosis. There is a noticeable loss of vocal resonance with nasal obstruction, but this is conspicuous when the maxillary antra are filled with fluid. As with fluid in the lung, for which the well-known change of sound on auscultation is diagnostic, a stethoscope held over the maxillary sinus will detect a similar alteration in sound transmission.

   Diagnostic ultrasound techniques have made use of this, and instruments are now available in which ultrasonic waves are directed into the antrum, and reflect differently when the sinus contains fluid. Ultrasound for the diagnosis of maxillary sinusitis has not become established, and x-rays remain a more reliable help in the diagnosis of sinusitis.

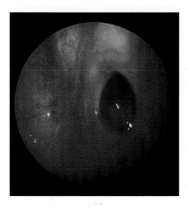

62 The ostium of the maxillary sinus as seen through the endoscope.

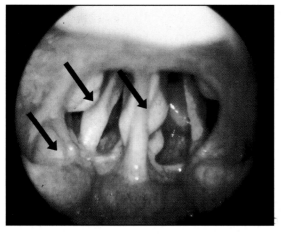

63 The post-nasal space seen with a fibreoptic endoscope. A panoramic view showing most of the anatomical features photographed through the fibreoptic endoscope (see **4**, **52**). *(Left arrow—* Eustachian orifice; *middle arrow—*posterior end of inferior turbinate; *right arrow—*posterior border of septum.)

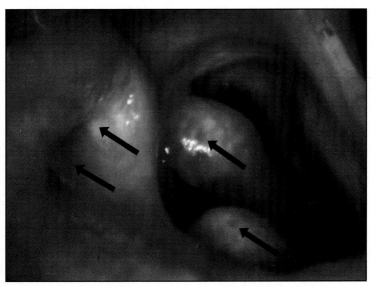

64 The post-nasal space. Enlarged view of **63** to show the Eustachian orifice and posterior ends of the middle and inferior turbinate.

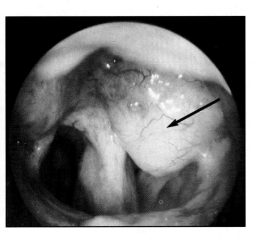

65 A post-nasal cyst (Thornvaldts, *arrow*) demonstrated with a fibreoptic photograph of the post-nasal space.

EXAMINATION OF THE PHARYNX AND LARYNX

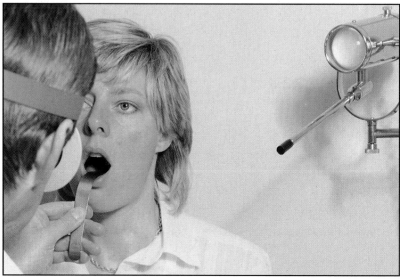

66 Examination of the pharynx. A tongue depressor is necessary to obtain a clear view of the tonsillar region.

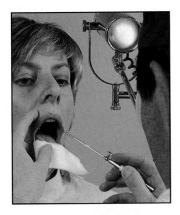

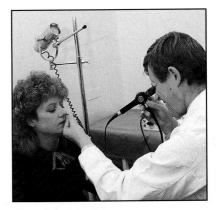

67 Examination of the larynx using the laryngeal mirror (indirect laryngoscopy). A good view of the larynx is obtained with most patients. The valleculae, pyriform fossae, arytenoids, ventricular bands and cords should all be clearly seen. It requires some inhibition of the gag reflex by the patient, and a local anaesthetic lozenge or spray may be necessary.

The tongue is held between the thumb and middle finger, and the upper lip retracted with the index finger. This examination is difficult in children, not only because they may be uncooperative, but because the infantile epiglottis is curved, unlike the 'flat' adult epiglottis, and occludes a clear view of the larynx. Therefore, direct laryngoscopy under anaesthetic is usually necessary to diagnose the cause of hoarseness in a child.

Fibreoptic laryngoscopy is a further technique for seeing the difficult larynx.

68 Fibreoptic endoscopy of the upper respiratory tract. When the post-nasal space and larynx are difficult to see with routine mirror examination, the fibreoptic endoscope, which can be inserted through the nose, gives a view of the nasal fossae, post-nasal space and the larynx. A topical anaesthetic is used on the nasal mucosa before the endoscope is introduced. The field is small, however, and one has to be experienced in the use fibreoptic endoscopes to be confident of excluding pathology in the larynx. A small television camera may be attached to the endoscope so that a large view may be seen on the TV monitor.

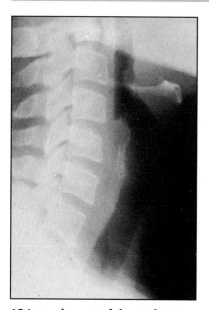

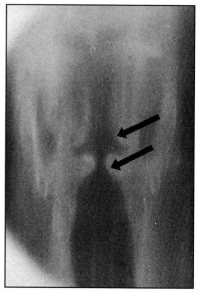

69 Lateral x-ray of the neck. A lateral x-ray of the neck gives helpful information about the anatomy of the base of the tongue, larynx, trachea and upper oesophagus. The upper oesophagus is normally approximately the width of the trachea. An increase in the width of the oesophagus is suggestive of significant pathology needing further investigation, such as a barium swallow x-ray or oesophagoscopy.

70 Laryngeal tomogram. This shows the cords (*lower arrow*) and ventricular bands (*upper arrow*), and is used to confirm the site and extent of a lesion. Small lesions on the cord can be detected, and 'hidden sites' in the larynx, such as the ventricle and subglottic region, are well demonstrated. A CT scan also shows laryngeal anatomy.

TASTE AND SMELL

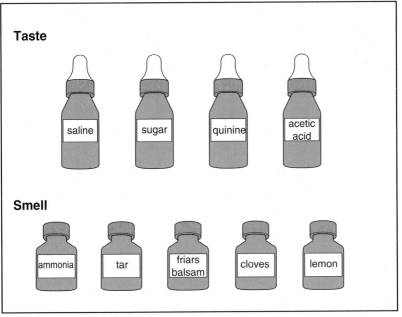

Taste

saline sugar quinine acetic acid

Smell

ammonia tar friars balsam cloves lemon

71 Solutions used to test taste and smell. Four solutions are used to test taste. The solution is placed on one side of the tongue and the patient is asked to identify the taste, whether sweet, salt, sour or bitter. This is a relatively crude qualitative test.

Testing for anosmia is done with a series of smell solutions for the patient to recognise.

1. This odour smells most like	2. This odour smells most like	3. This odour smells most like
a. petrol	a. tomato	a. whisky
b. pizza	b. liquorice	b. honey
c. peanuts	c. strawberry	c. lime
d. lilac	d. menthol	d. cherry

72 Anosmia 'scratch card' tests. A disc impregnated with a specific odour which is released when the disc is scratched with the fingernail; the smell identity is then marked on the card. Quantitative tests are not in routine clinical use, although 'olfactometers' with measured odours for smell assessment are described.

Anosmia may be a complication of fracture of the anterior cranial fossa. or it may follow influenza; recovery is uncommon. Temporary anosmia will occur with severe nasal obstruction.

Anosmia is invariably linked with a complaint of impaired taste; this is usually found to be normal on testing, and the sensation of smell is an adjunct to the full subtle appreciation of taste. The dependence on smell for taste appreciation varies from person to person, so that a complaint of taste loss may or may not accompany anosmia.

One is dependent on the integrity of the patient's response to smell and taste tests. It is, therefore, often impossible to be certain in medico-legal cases whether anosmia or ageusia is genuine. With smell, a failure to identify a very strong stimulus such as ammonia suggests malingering, as the Vth rather than the Ist cranial nerve is involved.

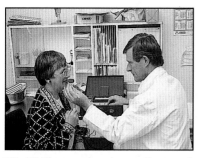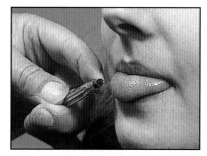

73, 74 Electrogustometry. Electricity has a metallic taste, and when a small current in micro-amps is applied to the tongue, a quantitative reading can be obtained. The normal threshold on the margin of the tongue is between 5 and 30 μa. This more refined test of taste is also of interest in conditions such as facial palsy or acoustic neuroma, in which the chorda tympani nerve may be involved.

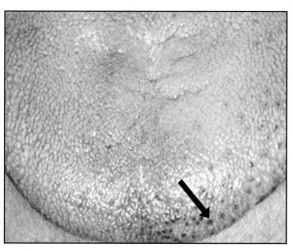

75 The taste buds. These are mainly situated on the tongue and palate, and are centred on the fungiform and circumvallate papillae. The **fungiform papillae** (*arrowed*) degenerate with age, and are prominent on a child's tongue. They also atrophy, as seen here, from the right side of the tongue to the mid-line, with the loss of the chorda tympani nerve, which may be divided in ear surgery.

The filiform papillae account for the rough surface of the tongue and are not related to the taste sensation.

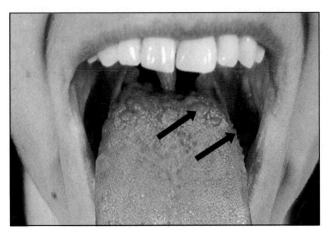

76 Circumvallate papillae. These are often prominent on the base of the tongue. A patient may be alarmed when looking at the tongue to notice these normal structures and mistake them for a serious disease, The foliate linguae on the margin of the tongue near the anterior pillar of the fauces may cause similar concern.

The *top arrow* indicates the circumvallate papillae. The *bottom arrow* points to the foliate linguae.

Chapter 2

The Ear

THE PINNA

DEFORMITIES

The pinna is formed from the coalescence of six tubercles and developmental abnormalities are common.

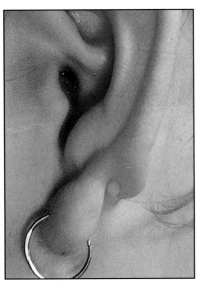

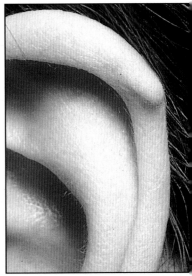

77 Minor deformities. These are of little importance. This shows duplication of the lobule.

78 Darwin's tubercle. A deformity of the pinna of phylogenetic interest. It is homologous to the tip of the mammalian ear and may be sufficiently prominent to justify surgical excision. Although Darwin's name is used for this tubercle, Woolmer gave the first description.

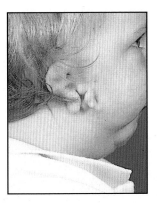

79 Microtia. Absence of the pinna or gross deformity is often associated with meatal atresia and ossicular abnormalities. Faulty development of the 1st and 2nd branchial arches results in aural deformities which may be associated with hypoplasia of the maxilla and mandible and eyelid deformities (Treacher–Collins syndrome, **84**). This type of pinna deformity is difficult to reconstruct.

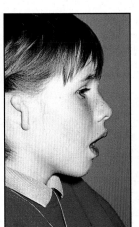
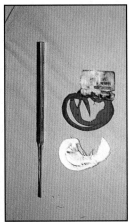
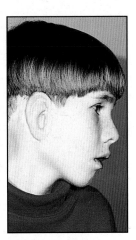

80–82 Surgical reconstruction for microtia. Multiple surgical procedures are usually necessary, and a near-normal pinna is difficult to achieve. Rib cartilage grafts are taken and fashioned to act as a scaffold for local skin rotation flaps and free skin grafts. The reconstruction is a challenge to the innovative surgeon and results vary with the severity of pinna deformity.

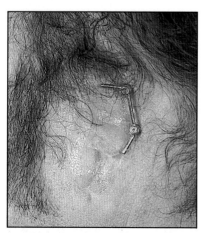 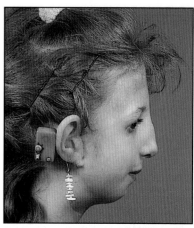

83, 84 Gross microtia with a bone-anchored prosthesis and hearing aid.
If microtia is gross, it may be better either to advise no treatment or a prosthesis rather than reconstruction. Prosthetic ears (**84**, right) have improved greatly in recent years, and it is now possible for these to be attached to the cranium using screws and plates (osseo-integrated implants) with a bone-anchored hearing aid.

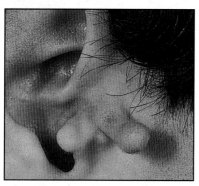 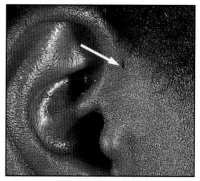

85 Hillocks (or accessory lobules).
These are commonly found anterior to the tragus, and are excised for cosmetic reasons. A small nodule of cartilage may be found underlying these hillocks.

86 Pre-auricular sinuses which are closely related to the anterior crus of the helix cause many problems. Discharge with recurrent swelling and inflammation may occur. The small opening of the sinus (*arrow*) is easily missed on examination, particularly when it is concealed, as may rarely be the case, behind the fold of the helix, rather than in the more obvious anterior site.

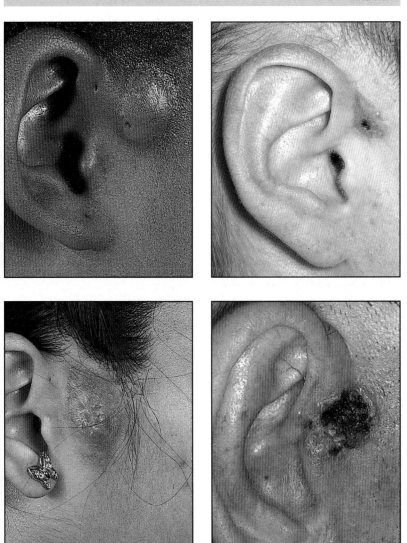

87–90 An infected pre-auricular sinus. A furuncle or skin ulceration in this site is diagnostic of an underlying infected pre-auricular sinus. Quite extensive skin loss can occur in this site with recurrent infection of a pre-auricular sinus.

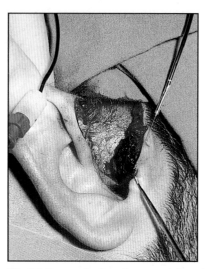 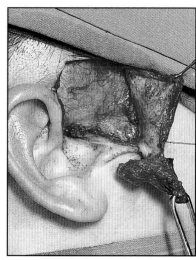

91, 92 Pre-auricular sinus excision. A furuncle or skin inflammation, which may be quite extensive in this pre-auricular site, is invariably related to a pre-auricular sinus. Careful examination for the sinus must be made.

Excision when the infection is quiescent is necessary and this, although minor surgery, is not easy. A long-branched and lobular structure must be excised. Incomplete excision of the tract leads to further infection and the need for revision surgery. To ensure complete excision of the pre-auricular sinus, the extension of an endaural incision as shown is needed, with reflection of the skin anteriorly down to the temporal facia.

If the sac is injected with a dye it is better defined, and it is possible to be certain of complete excision if the sac is dissected from its deep aspect towards the sinus punctum, which is excised with an elipse of skin.

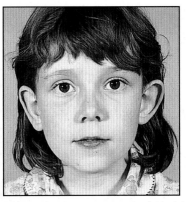 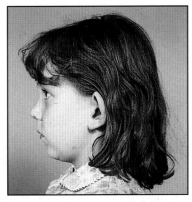

93, 94 Prominent ears. The fold of the antihelix is either absent or poorly formed in a prominent ear; it is not simply that the angle between the posterior surface of the conchal cartilage and the cranium is more 'open'. Parents and child may be offended by the diagnosis of Bat or Lop ears, although these terms are commonly used.

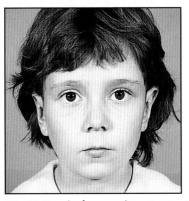 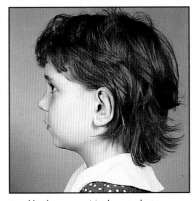

95, 96 Surgical correction aims to give a natural-looking ear. Modern techniques avoid a 'pinned back' appearance with a sharp, tender antihelix. Re-shaping of the cartilage of the pinna is necessary, and recurrence follows simple excision of post-auricular skin.

Prominent ears are best corrected between the ages of four and six years at the beginning of school, but there is no additional surgical problem in correcting adult ears. Youngsters may be the subject of considerable ridicule in early years because of Bat ears and, therefore, surgical correction is not to be deferred.

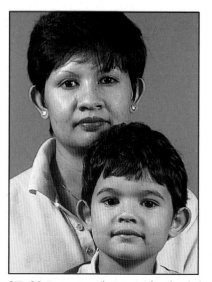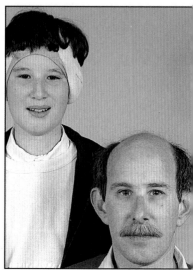

97, 98 Bat ears. These are often familial. Approximately 60% of bat ears are noted at, or soon after, birth. In the first six months of life, the ear cartilage may be moulded and correction of prominent ears may be achieved by splinting. Surgery is the only remedy thereafter. The son (**98**, right) has the firm ear dressing required for 5–10 days after operation for prominent ears.

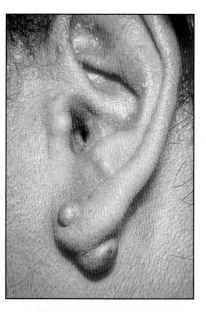

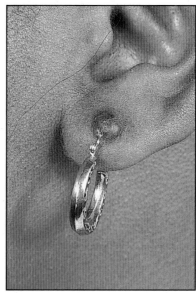

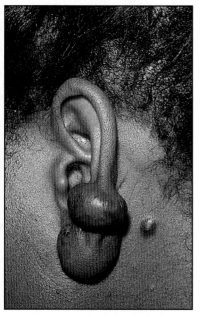

99–101 Keloid formation is common in black people, and is difficult to treat. Recurrence follows excision, and repeated excision may lead to huge keloid formation. Radiotherapy or local triamcinolone injections following excision reduce the incidence of recurrence of the keloid. Pressure at the site of keloid excision has also been shown to reduce recurrence. Special pressure clip-on ear-rings are available to apply to the ear lobe after operation. Keloid formation is common near the ear and on the neck, but is almost **unheard of in the middle third of the face**.

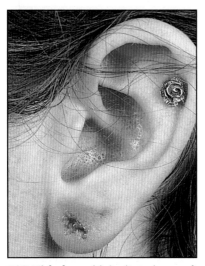

102 Nickel sensitivity limits the use of certain ear-rings.

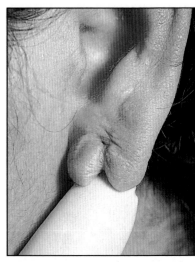

103 Trauma. Traumatic 'cutting-out' when the ear-ring is pulled by a baby or adult in ill-humour. Infection at the time the sleepers are inserted is another hazard.

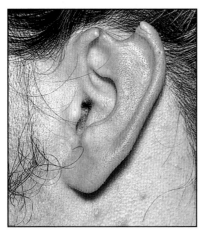

104 Trauma to the pinna. The projecting and obvious pinna is a frequent site for trauma. Partial or complete avulsion is common. This loss of tissue is from a bite.

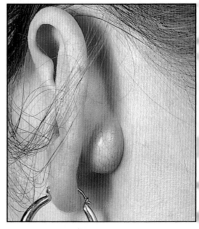

105 A Sebaceous cyst near the site of an ear-ring puncture. The punctum is just apparent and is diagnostic. Sebaceous cysts are common behind the ear, particularly in the post-aural sulcus.

107

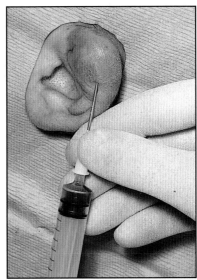

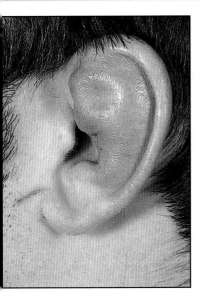

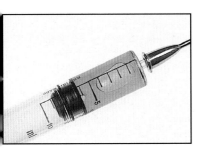

106–108 Haematomas of the pinna following trauma. Bruising with minimal swelling settles. A haematoma or collection of serous fluid, however, is common, and these, particularly if recurrent from frequent injury and left untreated, will result in a 'cauliflower ear'. The fluid, if aspirated with a syringe (**107** and **108**), usually recurs, and incision and drainage may be necessary. Some thickening, however, of the underlying cartilage invariably takes place, and a return to a completely normal-shaped pinna is not usual.

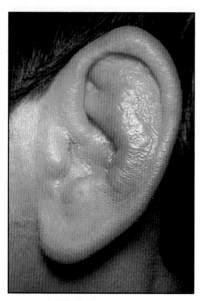

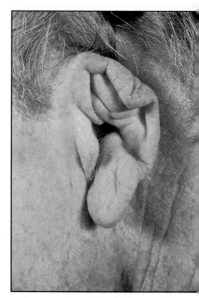

109 Perichondritis. A painful red and swollen pinna accompanied by fever, following trauma or surgery, suggests an infection of the cartilage. The organism is frequently ***Pseudomonas pyocyanea***.

110 Collapse of the pinna cartilage following perichondritis. This happened prior to the availability of effective antibiotics. However, perichondritis is still a worrying complication which requires intensive antibiotic treatment.

Collapsing or alteration of the shape of the pinna cartilage may also occur in relapsing polychondritis.

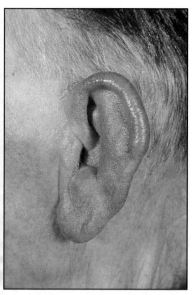

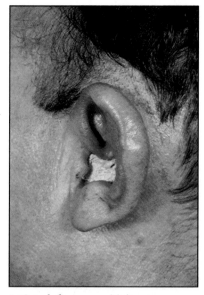

111 Relapsing polychondritis. This
is a rare inflammatory condition involving
destruction and replacement with fibrous
tissue of body cartilage. In this case, the
elastic aural cartilage has been replaced
by fibrous tissue so that the ear has an
unusual 'felty' feel and does not have any
'spring' on palpation.

The larynx cartilage also may be
affected, causing hoarseness which may
proceed to stridor. The nasal septum may
collapse. One or more of the lower limb
joints are usually swollen and painful.

112 Iodoform sensitivity. An
antiseptic ear dressing commonly used
contains bismuth, iodoform and paraffin
(B.I.P.). Sensitivity to iodoform may occur,
and a red ear with marked irritation
suggests this complication (rather than
perichondritis, which is characterised by
pain). Neomycin is one of the more
commonly used topical antibiotics that
may give rise to a skin sensitivity.

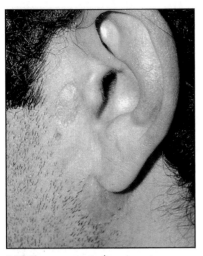

113 Burn scars in the ear region are evidence of the past use of cautery to relieve ear symptoms in childhood. In the Arab world, these burns are still common, and are known as chowes.

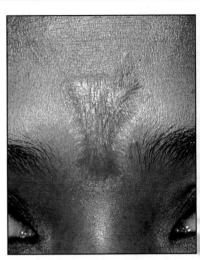

114 A chowe in the mid-forehead where burn treatment was used in the past for headache.

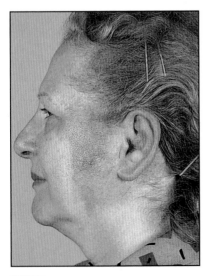

115 Erysipelas is caused by haemolytic streptococci entering fissures in the skin near the orifice of the ear meatus (fissures such as those in otitis externa).

A well-defined, raised erythema spreads to involve the face. This condition, which is often accompanied by malaise and fever, was serious in the pre-antibiotic era, but settles rapidly with penicillin.

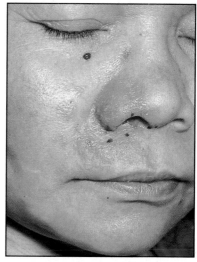

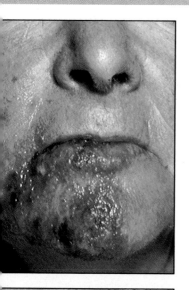

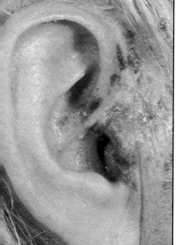

116–118 The herpes zoster virus in the head and neck may affect the gasserian ganglion of the Vth cranial nerve. Here the mandibular (**116**) and the maxillary (**117**) divisions are involved.

The vesicular type of skin eruption is confined to the distribution of the nerve. The ophthalmic division of V is most frequently involved, but all three divisions of V are rarely affected at the same time. The herpes zoster virus also involves the geniculate ganglion of the VIIth cranial nerve (***Ramsay–Hunt syndrome or geniculate herpes***). Herpes affects the pinna and pre-auricular region (**118**), and is associated with a facial palsy. In most cases, there is also vertigo and sensori-neural deafness. There is less likelihood of a full recovery of the facial palsy than in Bell's palsy.

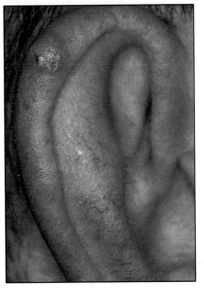

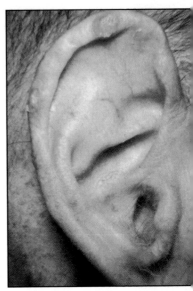

119 Basal-cell carcinoma. Ulcers on the helix are common. A long history suggests a basal-cell carcinoma. This is treated with wedge resection. An ulcer of short duration suggests a squamous-cell carcinoma or more rarely a melanoma, both of which require more extensive surgical resection.

120 Solar keratoses. These warty growths affect the skin of the fair-headed when exposed to strong sunlight. They may become malignant. The skin of the helix may be affected with several of these keratoses.

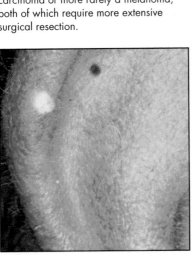

121 Gouty tophi form a characteristic lesion on the helix.

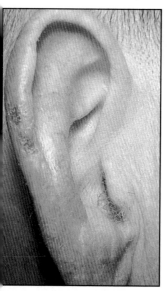

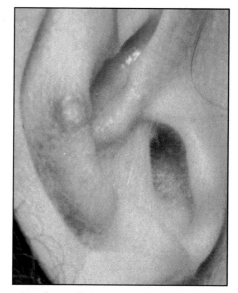

122 Inflammatory ulcers.
These affect the helix and occasion-ally the antihelix. The lesions on the helix are blessed with a lengthy diagnosis—***chondro-dermatitis nodularis helicis chronicis***, which presents as a long-standing intermittent ulceration. It is primarily a chronic chondritis with secondary skin infection. A wedge resection of the ulcer and cartilage may be necessary, as the ulcer only heals temporarily with ointments.

123 Ulcers of the antihelix. These are usually traumatic (on a particularly prominent antihelix fold) and are primarily a skin lesion. A basal or squamous-cell carcinoma, however, may present on the antihelix.

THE EXTERNAL AUDITORY MEATUS

The skin of the external auditory meatus is migratory and does not desquamate.

Cleaning of the ear canal is therefore unnecessary—those who diligently clean their ears, or those of their children, with cotton buds etc, hinder the migration of skin, and wax tends to accumulate, causing otitis externa to develop.

Some people have non-migratory skin of the external auditory meatus and are susceptible to episodes of otitis externa. The meatuses tend to become occluded with desquamated skin wax and debris, and periodic cleaning of the ears is necessary. The migration of meatal epithelium is also abnormal in keratosis obturans. In this condition, desquamated epithelium accumulates and may form a large impacted mass in the meatus, causing erosion of the bony canal.

In the past, skin grafts initially used for myringoplasty often failed or led to otitis externa, because skin taken from elsewhere on the body did not take on this migratory role; fascia is now used to graft the ear drum.

Although wax normally does not accumulate because of meatal skin migration, it may impact and cause a hearing loss, which may necessitate syringing.

124

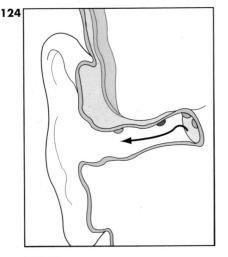

124–128 A migrating ink dot. A dot of ink, if placed near the centre of the drum (**124,125**), is found to lie near the margin of the drum after 3 weeks (**126**), and between 6–12 weeks the dot migrates outwards on the meatal skin (**127** and **128**) to emerge in wax at the orifice of the meatus.

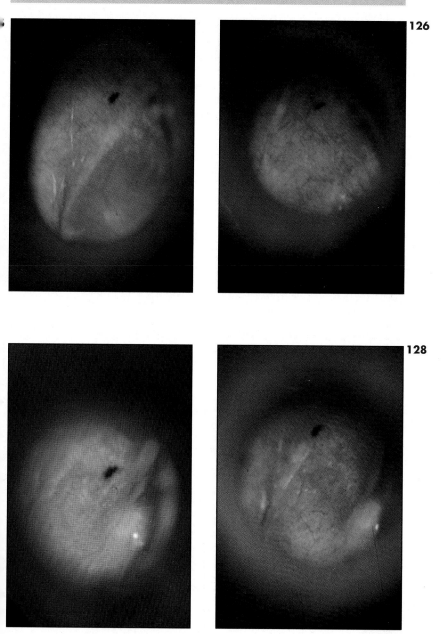

126

128

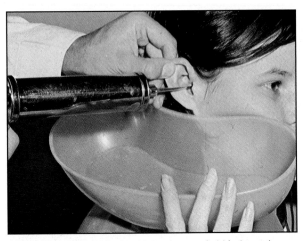

129 Syringing. The rather large syringe of old-fashioned appearance has changed little in the past 100 years, and remains a simple and effective treatment for wax impaction. The pinna is pulled outwards and backwards to straighten the meatus, and water at body temperature is irrigated along the posterior wall of the ear. The water finds a passage past the wax, rebounds off the drum and pushes the wax outwards. Hard wax may require the use of drops before syringing.

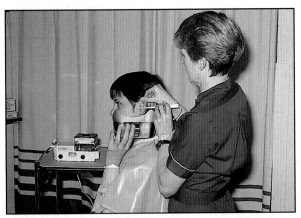

130 A modern ear syringe with an electronically operated pump.

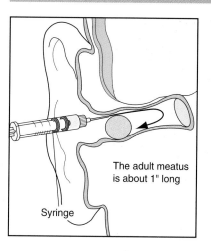

131 Syringing of the ear.

The adult meatus
is about 1" long

Syringe

Syringing is not painful, therefore pain means either an error in technique or that there is an otitis externa or a perforation. If there is a perforation, the ear should not be syringed; pain with vertigo may occur with subsequent otitis media and otorrhoea, and a past history of discharge suggests a perforation. Coughing (from the vagal reflex—the auricular branch of the vagus supplies the drum) or syncope may complicate syringing. Vertigo with nystagmus will occur if the water is too hot or too cold.

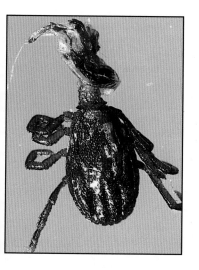

132 An insect foreign body in the ear. The insect was adherent to the tympanic membrane, giving a sensation of discomfort and a deceptive drum appearance on examination; this insect was removed with syringing.

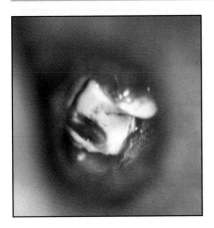

133 Foreign body in the ear.

The main danger of a foreign body in the ear lies in its careless removal.

Syringing is very effective and safe for small metallic foreign bodies. Vegetable foreign bodies, such as peas, swell with water and are better not syringed. Insects not uncommonly become impacted in the meatus, particularly in the tropics. Maggots cause a painful ear, and their removal is difficult; insufflation of calomel powder is usually effective treatment.

Previous attempts to remove a piece of plastic wedged in the child's meatus have led to bleeding in the meatus. The drum against which the foreign body impinges can be seen deep to the plastic.

One must not persevere in attempts to remove an aural foreign body, particularly in a child, as a perforation is easily caused. If immediate removal with a hook or syringe is not effective, the patient must be admitted for removal under general anaesthetic with the help of the microscope. It is often dangerous to use forceps to remove an aural foreign body, since the object easily slips from the jaws of the forceps to go deeper into the meatus.

Otitis externa

Eczema of the meatus and pinna (as in **134**) may be associated with eczema elsewhere, particularly in the scalp, or it may be an isolated condition affecting only one ear. *Itching* is the main symptom, with scanty discharge. The eczematous type of otitis externa usually settles with cleaning of the meatus, followed by the use of a topical corticosteroid and antibiotic, but recurrence is common.

The patient should avoid over-diligent cleaning of the meatus or scratching the ear, and should prevent water entering the meatus during washing or swimming, as these are some of the factors predisposing to recurrence.

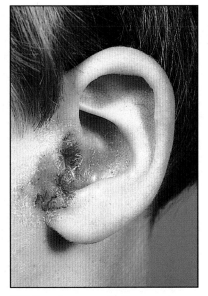

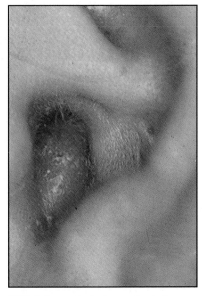

134 Ear drop sensitivity may worsen an otitis externa. Chloramphenicol drops caused this condition. Neomycin less commonly causes similar reactions.

Patients should be advised to discontinue ear drops that cause an increase in irritation or are painful.

135 A furuncle in the meatus is the other common type of otitis externa. It is characterised by pain; pain on movement of the pinna or on inserting the auriscope is diagnostic of a furuncle. Diabetes mellitus must be excluded with recurrent furuncles.

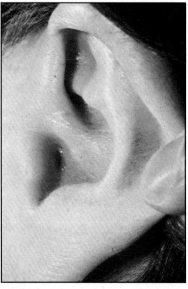

136 Furunculosis. This is a generalised infection of the meatal skin. Pain is severe and the canal is narrowed or occluded so that examination with the auriscope is extremely painful and no view of the deep meatus is possible. A swab of the pus should be taken, and treatment is with systemic antibiotics and a meatal dressing (e.g. glycerine and ichthyol, or a corticosteroid cream with an antibiotic). The organism may be transferred by the patient's finger from the nasal vestibules, and a nasal swab is a relevant investigation, particularly with recurrent furuncles.

The lymph nodes adjacent to the pinna are enlarged with a furuncle or furunculosis, and a tender mastoid node may mimic a cortical mastoid abscess.

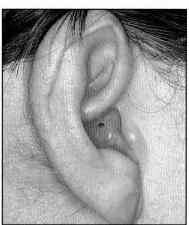

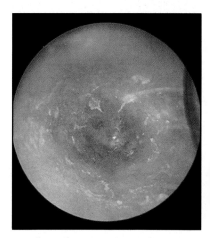

137,138 'Deep' otitis externa. An uncommon form of otitis externa involves predominantly the skin of the deep bony meatus and the surface of the tympanic membrane. The drum epithelium may become replaced with sessile granulations (**granular myringitis**) infected with *Pseudomonas pyocyanea*.

In protracted cases of this type of otitis externa, the skin of the deep meatus and drum becomes thickened and 'funnelled' with meatal atresia. The resulting conductive hearing loss is extremely difficult to treat surgically once this condition is quiescent.

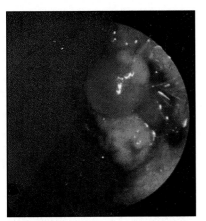

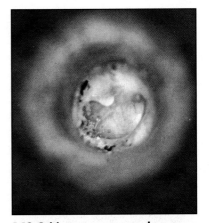

139 'Malignant' otitis externa is a rare and serious form of otitis externa to which elderly diabetics are particularly susceptible. Granulation tissue is found in the meatus infected with *Pseudomonas* and anaerobic organisms. This granulation tissue tends to erode deeply, involving the middle and inner ear, the bone of the skull base with extension to the brain and also the great vessels of the neck. The condition is therefore frequently fatal.

Intense antibiotic therapy often associated with surgical drainage of the affected areas is necessary. It is not a 'malignant' condition in the histological sense, for the biopsies of granulation tissue show inflammatory changes only; 'necrotizing' otitis externa may be more adequate, but 'malignant' indicates the serious clinical nature.

140 Otitis externa secondary to discharge via a drum perforation is initially treated (an ear swab having been taken for culture and sensitivity) with cleaning of the meatus and the instillation of the appropriate antibiotic and cortico-steroid drops. If the condition persists with marked irritation and pain, a ***fungal otitis externa*** should be suspected. In persistent infection, the meatus contains a cocktail of drops, pus and desquamated skin. In fungal infections, as shown here, the dark spores of *Aspergillus niger* and white mycelium of *Candida albicans* can be seen. Thorough cleaning of the meatus precedes treatment with a topical antifungal agent.

The meatal skin infection is introduced from outside—usually from the patient's finger, or from water, particularly after swimming.

The infection, however, may be from the middle ear if there is a perforation, and discharge from chronic otitis media may be the cause of a persistent otitis externa.

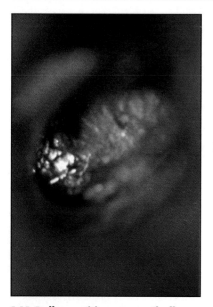

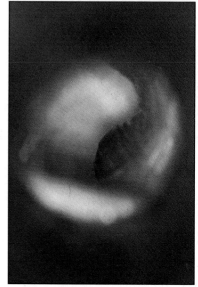

141 Bullous otitis externa (bullous myringitis). This unusual otitis externa frequently follows influenza or an upper respiratory tract infection. A complaint of earache followed by bleeding, then followed by relief of pain is diagnostic of this condition.

Examination shows haemorrhagic blebs on the drum and meatus, similar to the vesicular eruption of herpes. If there is pyrexia with a conductive hearing loss, the otitis externa is associated with an otitis media, and systemic antibiotics are necessary. In the absence of pyrexia and hearing loss, this condition settles spontaneously without treatment.

142 Otitis externa with herpes zoster. Otitis externa occurs with herpes zoster involving either the gasserian or geniculate ganglion, and the vesicles may be haemorrhagic.

Carcinomas and melanomas in the skin of the external auditory meatus are rare, but any persistent granulation or skin lesion should be biopsied.

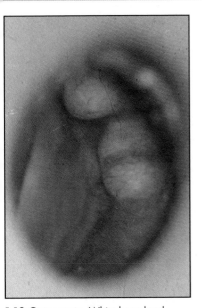 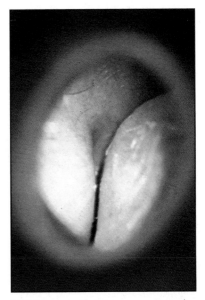

143 Osteomas. White bony hard swellings in the deep meatus are a common finding during a routine examination. They usually remain small and symptom free, and tend to be symmetrical in both ears.

Swimmers are susceptible to these lesions, which are sometimes called '*swimmer's osteomas*'. There is experimental evidence to show that irrigation of the bony meatus with cold water produces a periostitis that leads to osteoma formation. Histologically, these bony lesions are hyperostosis, rather than a bony tumour, so that the term 'osteoma', although established, is not strictly correct.

144 Large osteomas may narrow the meatus to a chink so that wax accumulates and is difficult to syringe. Otitis externa is also a complication.

These osteomas, therefore, may require surgical removal with a microdrill. They should not be removed with a gouge, for a fracture with bleeding in the remaining osteoma is a probable complication, causing damage to the facial nerve and resulting in facial palsy.

It is rare for osteomas to occlude the meatus completely, and in almost all cases no treatment is required.

THE TYMPANIC MEMBRANE AND MIDDLE EAR

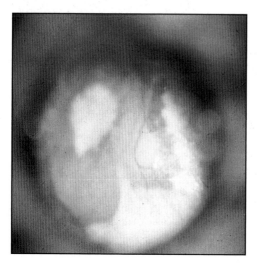

145 'Chalk' patches. White areas of ***tympanosclerosis*** are common findings on examination of the drum. They are of little significance in themselves, and the hearing is often normal. A past history of otorrhoea in childhood is usual, but chalk patches do occur with no apparent past otitis media.

Extensive tympanosclerosis with a rigid drum is a sequela of past otitis media, and the ossicles, too, may be fixed or non-continuous.

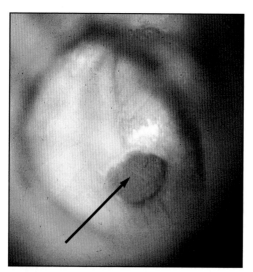

146 Scarring of the drum. A gossamer-thin membrane can be seen to close this previously well-defined central perforation (*arrow*). At first sight with the auriscope, a central perforation would appear to be the diagnosis; more careful examination with a pneumatic otoscope will show that this thin membrane moves and seals the defect, giving reassurance that the drum is intact.

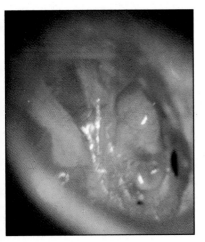 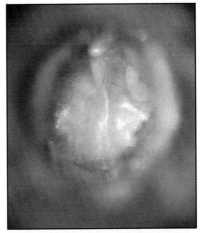

147 Scarring of the drum. Scarring of the drum with retraction onto the promontory, incus and round window is also evidence of past otitis media. It is sometimes difficult to be sure whether this type of drum is intact; a thin layer of epithelium indrawn on to the middle ear structures may seal the middle ear, and examination with the operating microscope may be necessary to be certain of an intact drum.

148 Scarred tympanic membrane. A scarred tympanic membrane in which the drum has become atelectatic and indrawn onto the long process of the incus, promontory and round window.

149

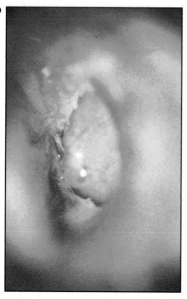

149–151 Traumatic perforation. A blow on the ear with the hand is a common cause of traumatic perforation which has an irregular margin, and there is fresh blood or blood clot on the drum. The defect is frequently slit-shaped (**151**). Pain and transient vertigo at the time of injury are followed by a tinnitus and hearing loss.

150

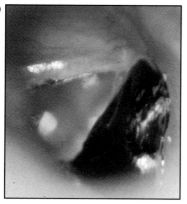
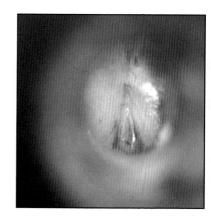

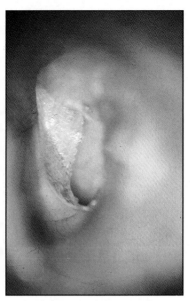

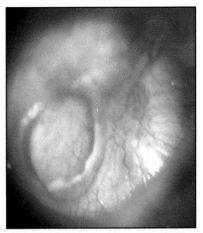

153 Central perforation. Acute otitis media with pus under pressure in the middle ear may rupture the drum, and although healing usually occurs, a permanent perforation can result. These perforations are usually central. A small perforation may be symptom-free, but episodes of otorrhoea with head colds and after swimming are common, along with a conductive hearing loss.

The otorrhoea tends to be profuse and muco-purulent, and may be intermittent or persistent. This type of central perforation, when dry, is successfully closed with a fascial graft (myringoplasty). Other complications with central perforations are rare, so they are described as **'safe' perforations**. A central perforation may persist after an episode of acute otitis media and otorrhoea in childhood; myringoplasty is usually delayed in children since closure by puberty is common. If, however, the upper respiratory tract is free of infection, and the perforation is the site of recurrent infections with impaired hearing, these are indications to proceed with myringoplasty in childhood.

152 Healing perforation. Almost all traumatic perforations heal spontaneously within two months, a thin membrane growing across the defect.

Traumatic perforations are usually central, but if the perforation extends to the annulus, healing may not occur. The extremely large traumatic perforations may also fail to close spontaneously.

Taking care to avoid water entering the middle ear and avoiding inflating the middle ear with the Valsalva manoeuvre are the only precautions the patient need take.

A middle-ear infection with discharge is the commonest complication, usually settling with a course of topical and systemic antibiotics. Blast injuries, barotrauma, foreign bodies or their careless removal, and even over-enthusiastic kissing of the ear may also cause traumatic perforations.

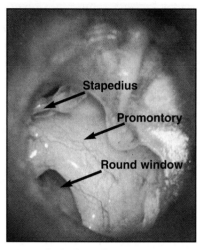

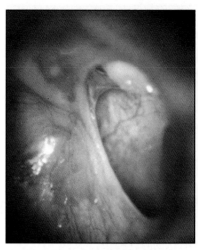

154 Marginal perforation. A perforation may reach the annulus posteriorly and is called marginal. The middle-ear structures are frequently seen through the perforation. The well-defined margin of the round window is particularly obvious, and the promontory, incudostapedial joint and stapedius are also apparent.

155 Squamous epithelium on the incus. The marginal perforation may enable squamous epithelium to migrate into the middle ear. In this ear, white squamous epithelium has formed on the incus. Marginal perforations, therefore, are described as **'unsafe'** since there is a risk of cholesteatoma.

Perforations of the pars flaccida (attic perforations) are invariably associated with cholesteatoma formation.

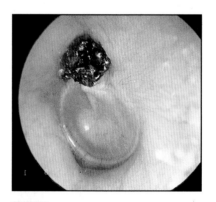

156 Attic perforation. Debris adherent to the pars flaccida of the drum suggests an underlying attic perforation.

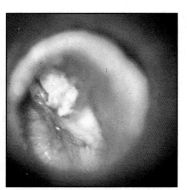

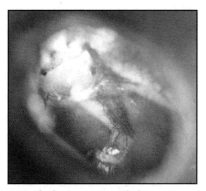

157 Cholesteatoma. The debris, when removed, exposes a white mass of epithelium characteristic of a cholesteatoma. Cholesteatoma is not a neoplasm; it is simply squamous epithelium in the middle ear.

If ignored, it increases in size, becomes infected and is associated with a scanty fetid otorrhoea. It may erode bone, leading to serious complications: extension to involve the dura with intracranial infection may occur, and the facial nerve and labyrinth too may be eroded. The **extent** of the cholesteatoma determines the danger: a small attic pocket of epithelium is relatively harmless, and can be removed with suction, but an extensive mass of epithelium is dangerous and needs exploration and removal via a mastoidectomy approach.

A chronic discharging ear is not painful, and persistent pain and headache, or severe vertigo, strongly suggest an intracranial complication or labyrinthitis.

158 Cholesteatoma. Cholesteatoma erodes the bony wall of the deep meatus so that a pocket containing white debris forms in the posterior-superior aspect of the drum.

The complete aetiology of the cholesteatoma is not understood. Migration of epithelium into the middle ear via an attic or posterior marginal perforation certainly accounts for most cholesteatomas. However, cholesteatoma may occur behind an intact drum, and may form with central perforations. Eustachian tube dysfunction with a negative pressure in the middle ear, if long-standing, leads to a chronic middle-ear effusion (chronic secretory otitis media) and a retracted drum. The pars flaccida retracts and may give the opportunity for a pocket of cholesteatoma to develop. In this picture of cholestea-toma, the remainder of the drum is a golden colour and fluid is present in the middle ear. The secretory otitis media may have been responsible for this cholesteatoma formation.

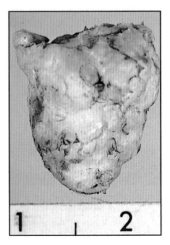

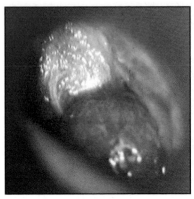

159 A cholesteatoma of 2 cm width removed at mastoidectomy presents the typical well-defined mass of white epithelium. The bone erosion that this mass causes shows on mastoid x-rays and CT or MRI scans.

160 Aural granulation. In the same way that epithelium may migrate through a perforation into the middle ear, mucous membrane may extrude out-wards to the meatus. Middle-ear mucous membrane extruding through a perfora-tion becomes infected and presents with a discharging ear. An aural granulation is seen in the deep meatus. Granulation may also form on the drum at the margin of the perfora-tion, and rarely granula-tion tissue forms on an intact drum in otitis externa (granular myringitis).

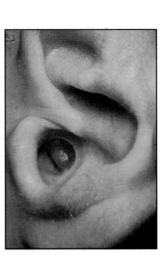

161 Pedunculated polyp. If the growth of granulation tissue is exuberant, a pedunculated polyp develops, which may present at the orifice of the meatus. Granulations and polyps commonly arise from the tympanic annulus posteriorly, but the originating site may also be the mucous membrane of the promontory, Eustachian tube orifice, and antrum and aditus.

Careful and thorough removal of polyps and granulation tissue to their site of origin is necessary. If the polyp is associated with cholesteatoma, removal by mastoid approach is required.

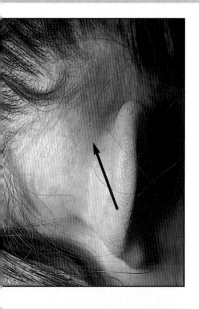

162 Mastoid abscess. A red, acutely tender swelling filling the post-auricular sulcus (*arrow*), and pushing the pinna conspicuously forwards and outwards, is characteristic of a mastoid abscess.

In the past, mastoidectomy was needed for an acute mastoid abscess complicating acute otitis media. This was extremely common in the pre-antibiotic era, and required exenteration of the mastoid air cells (***cortical mastoidectomy***). The operation is now rarely performed in countries where antibiotics are available.

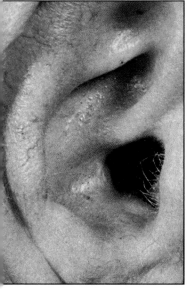

163 Enlarged meatus after mastoidectomy. A more extensive type of mastoidectomy is, however, still necessary for cholesteatoma which has extended beyond the middle ear.

This operation alters the anatomy of the ear. Examination after operation will show an enlarged meatus. At operation the meatus is enlarged with a meatoplasty to allow access to the mastoid cavity, so that wax can be removed with a Jobson–Horne probe or with suction. This is usually necessary once or twice a year, as the skin of the mastoid cavity does not migrate satisfactorily and therefore wax accumulates. Water entering in the ear following mastoidectomy should be avoided; infection and otorrhoea tend to follow. Syringing of a mastoid cavity is also to be avoided, not only because of the possibility of subsequent otorrhoea but because irrigation of water over the exposed lateral semi-circular canal causes vertigo.

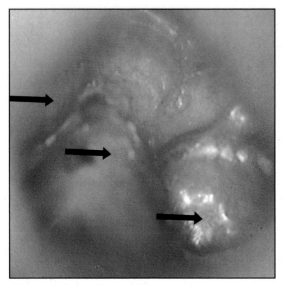

164 Auriscope view. With the auriscope, a ridge (containing the facial nerve) can be seen separating the drum anteriorly from the epithelized cavity posteriorly. Failure of the mastoid cavity to epithelize results in an infected cavity with discharge.

Top arrow points to the mastoid cavity; middle arrow indicates the facial ridge with the bone overlying the descending portion of the facial nerve; bottom arrow shows the tympanic membrane.

Surgical techniques aim to remove cholesteatoma without exteriorising the mastoid cavity, so that relatively normal anatomy is maintained post-operatively and hearing is maintained or improved (**intact canal wall tympanoplasty** although this operation is not suitable for every case. Although avoiding a mastoid cavity, the intact canal wall tympanoplasty technique tends to conceal recurrence of cholesteatoma. There are also surgical techniques to obliterate the mastoid cavity with muscle, fascia or bone grafts.

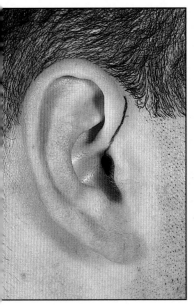 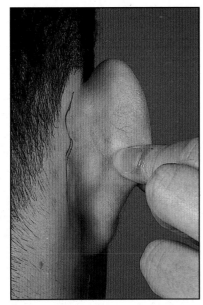

65, 166 Postaural and endaural incisions. These are two commonly used incisors for access to the middle ear and mastoid. The postaural is preferred if extensive mastoid exenteration is planned. The incision lines are delineated here, but in these sites the scars are imperceptible.

Otitis media with effusion (OME) or secretory otitis media

A sterile middle-ear exudate is a common cause of conductive hearing loss. It may occur when either a head cold or barotrauma interferes with Eustachian tube function, and it often follows acute otitis media. A post-nasal space neoplasm may also cause Eustachian tube obstruction, and is to be excluded in any adult with a persistent secretory otitis media.

In children, secretory otitis media is very common when adenoid tissue interferes with the Eustachian tube. The middle-ear fluid tends to be tenacious ('glue ear'), unlike the thin, straw-coloured exudate of adults.

The appearance of the drum is altered and the mobility reduced.

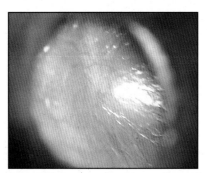 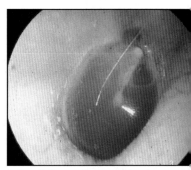

167, 168 Secretory otitis media with minimal drum change. The drum may look only slightly different, with a brown colour and some hyperaemia. A confident diagnosis of middle-ear fluid can only be made if reduced mobility is demonstrated and impedance audiometry (**35, 36**) is needed for confirmation.

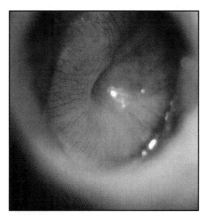

169 Secretory otitis media ('glue ear'). The colour change in this condition is often diagnostic, as well as the reduced mobility. The golden-brown colour showing through the translucent drum is readily apparent in the inferior part of this tympanic membrane.

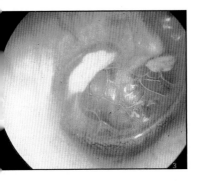

170 Secretory otitis media. A photograph with a fibreoptic camera gives a panoramic view of the deep meatus and membrane. Bubbles within the fluid and levels appearing as a hairline in the drum may be seen. A 'chalk' patch is also seen.

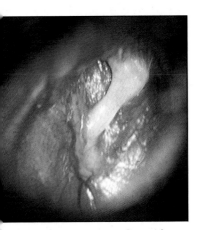

171 Secretory otitis media with marked drum change. The change is frequently gross, making the diagnosis obvious, with a golden colour, a retracted membrane and a prominent malleus.

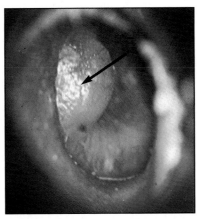

172 A vesicle on the drum (*arrow*) also occurs in children's glue ear.

The full aetiology of the Eustachian tube dysfunction causing secretory otitis media is at present unknown. Opinions therefore differ on the treatment, particularly that of children's 'glue ears'. Adenoid tissue in the region of the Eustachian tube orifice predisposes to 'glue ears', and adenoid removal is frequently necessary.

Glue ear

'Glue ear' is common between the ages of 3–6 years, and uncommonly persists after 11 years. The hearing loss is often slight and varies with colds. The self limiting nature of the condition calls for conservative treatment, but 'glue ears' are not to be ignored.

A marked and persistent hearing loss, interfering with schooling, necessitates surgery. Episodes of transient otalgia are common with 'glue ears', and frequent attacks of acute otitis media may occur. The drum may also become retracted and flaccid with prolonged middle-ear fluid. These features may necessitate the insertion of a grommet to reventilate the middle ear.

It is doubtful whether antihistamine and decongestant medicines, particularly in the absence of upper respiratory tract symptoms, have any influence on the course of 'glue ear'.

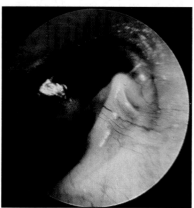

173 Blue drum. The middle-ear effusion evidently alters in composition, for at some stages in secretory otitis media the drum appears blue in colour—the so-called *'blue drum'*.

A similarly blue appearance of the tympanic membrane is seen following injury when bleeding occurs in the middle ear (haemotympanum). The conductive hearing loss associated with this injury resolves with resorption of the middle-ear haematoma. A persisting conductive hearing loss following injury, however, suggests injury to the ossicles with an ossicular discontinuity (see **186**).

Secretory otitis media may settle spontaneously. Nasal vasoconstrictor drops with an oral decongestant (an antihistamine with a pseudoephedrine preparation) may help recovery when there is associated upper respiratory tract allergy or infection. Insufflation of the Eustachian tube, either by the patient performing the Valsalva manoeuvre, Politzerisation or Eustachian catheterisation, may also influence recovery, but is not widely used.

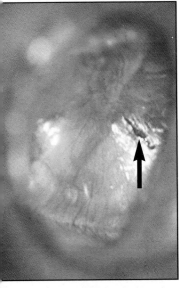

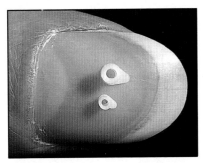

175 Grommets. The insertion of a grommet, a flanged teflon tube, is frequently needed to avoid a recurrence of middle-ear fluid.

174 Myringotomy. If secretory otitis media with poor hearing persists for over three months, myringotomy (under general anaesthetic in children), with aspiration of the fluid is often necessary.

Arrows indicate the radial incision of the myringotomy into which the grommet may be inserted. The posterior/superior quadrant of the drum is not used to avoid injury to the underlying incus and stapes.

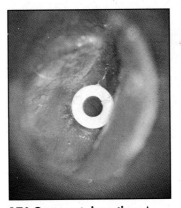

176 Grommet insertion. A myringotomy incision in the poster-ior half of the drum may damage the incudostapedial joint or round window, and a grommet inserted posteriorly may cause incus necrosis from pressure on the long process: an anterior or inferior radial myringotomy is a safer incision.

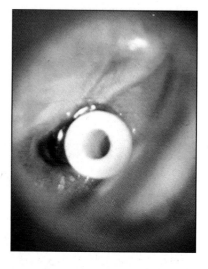

177 A grommet in place. The grommet tube ventilates the middle ear and acts instead of the Eustachian tube. Hearing and the appearance of the drum both return to normal.

The grommet usually extrudes spontaneously between 6–18 months to leave an intact drum, and is found in wax in the meatus. With recurrent middle-ear fluid, repeated grommet insertion may be needed. If normal Eustachian tube function has not returned and secretory otitis media recurs, the grommet is replaced.

Tympanosclerosis and drum scarring may ensue. This complication is also seen in untreated 'glue' ear. Minimal surgical trauma during grommet insertion is advisable. However, with a narrow ear canal, grommet insertion is not always technically easy.

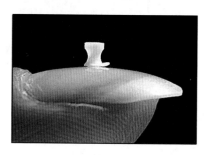

178 A mini-grommet causes less drum trauma, but extrusion is more rapid.

Obstruction of the Eustachian tube is a common and frequently diagnosed disorder. Abnormal patency of the tube (*the patulous Eustachian tube*) however, is also not uncommon, but the diagnosis is frequently missed.

The condition tends to occur in people who have lost weight or women who are taking 'the pill' or are pregnant. The symptoms are of a sensation of blockage in the ear, with normal hearing or minimal loss. Patients may comment that they hear themselves breathe and eat, and hear their own voice 'echo' in their ear. This sensation may alter with head movement (wrongly suggesting middle-ear fluid) and often is absent on lying down. Fortunately the symptoms are usually minor and settle spontaneously. Reassurance and explanation suffice as treatment in most cases. Failure to make the diagnosis, however, and treatment of the condition as Eustachian tube obstruction is common.

Chronic secretory otitis media

Middle-ear fluid, if persistent, may cause permanent changes in the drum. A secretory otitis media can cause hearing loss for decades, and the diagnosis is frequently overlooked in a long-standing hearing loss. Impedance audiometry helps in diagnosis.

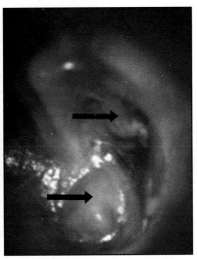

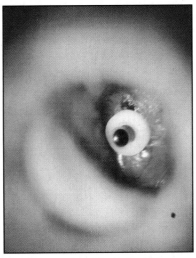

179 Grossly altered drum. A brown colour, with retraction of a flaccid membrane onto the ossicles and promontory, is seen with long-standing middle ear fluid. *Bottom arrow* points to indrawn drum onto the promontory; *top arrow* shows incudostapedial joint.

180 Grommet occluded with exudate. Insertion of a grommet in these chronic adult cases may restore hearing, but frequently either the lumen of the grommet becomes occluded with exudate, which may extrude through the tube into the meatus, or a constant otorrhoea occurs.

There is no present successful treatment for chronic secretory otitis media when this fails to respond to insertion of a grommet. A further problem with chronic secretory otitis media is the return of middle-ear fluid with hearing loss when the grommet extrudes. A larger flanged grommet, which remains in position longer, and periodic replacement are the present remedies.

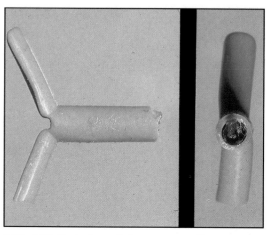 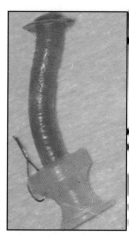

181, 182 Occlusion of the grommet lumen. Excess bleeding at the time of insertion may cause this problem, or subsequent occlusion with serous exudate. There are various designs of grommet or ventilation tube, and this Y-shaped tube shows the narrow lumen to be occluded.

Acute otitis media

Earache with conductive hearing loss and fever accompanying a head cold characterize acute otitis media. The drum is red and the landmarks are obscured; drum distension and pulsation may be seen.

Otitis media is common in children, probably due to their short, wide, Eustachian tube and the presence of adenoids which may be infected near the orifice. Rupture of the tympanic membrane in acute otitis media is not uncommon, and muco-purulent otorrhoea ensues with a pulsatile discharge. Penicillin is invariably curative, and complications are rare.

The middle-ear infection frequently settles without otorrhoea, but if the drum does rupture, a pulsating muco-purulent discharge filling the meatus is diagnostic of otitis media. A swab for culture and sensitivity is taken in these cases, although the ear usually becomes dry within 48 hours of penicillin therapy, and the perforation closes in most cases with little or no scarring.

Acute mastoiditis, previously serious and common, is almost unheard of where antibiotics are available. Myringotomy and cortical mastoidectomy are operations of the past for acute otitis media.

Secretory otitis media after the acute attack is the main complication today.

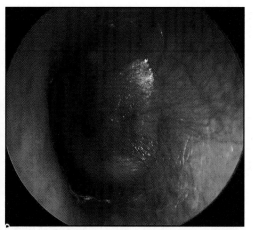

183 Acute otitis media
with bulging and hyperaemia of the posterior-superior quadrant of the tympanic membrane. This is the typical early appearance of acute otitis media photographed with a fibreoptic camera.

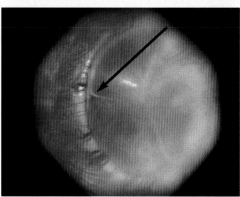

184 Glomus jugulare tumour. A photograph, via the fibreoptic endoscope, showing a glomus jugulare tumour presenting, as is characteristic, with a hyperaemia in the lower half of the drum. Middle-ear fluid is often present, and a meniscus is also seen (*arrow*).

The histology of a glomus jugulare tumour is similar to the carotid body tumour, with which it may co-exist. If the glomus tumour occupies the middle ear, it can be removed via a tympanotomy or mastoidectomy approach. When the jugular foramen is involved with loss of the IXth, Xth and XIth cranial nerve (often the XIIth from the anterior condylar foramen is also affected), the treatment is difficult. A surgical approach to the skull base is needed via the mastoid and neck, with a neurosurgical exposure if there is an intracranial extension.

If the tumour is surgically inaccessible, radiotherapy does slow the growth of an already very slow-growing tumour, and has an important place in the management, particularly in the more elderly patient. Microembolism under radiographic control of the vessels supplying the tumour is a further modality used in the treatment of these very vascular lesions, prior to surgery.

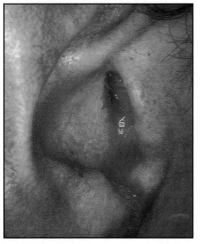

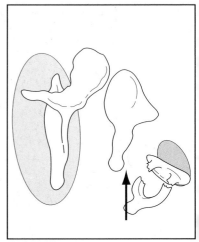

185 Bleeding. Bleeding from the ear or a red or 'blue' drum (see **173**), if the tympanic membrane does not rupture, may also follow a base-of-skull fracture with bleeding into the middle ear.

186 Injury to the ear ossicles. This may follow head injury. Dislocation of the incudostapedial joint is commonest (approximately 75%), but fracture of the stapes crura and disruption of the stapes footplate also occur.

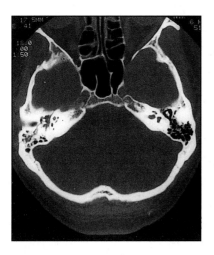

187 Skull fracture. Base-of-skull fracture involving the temporal bone, demonstrated on a CT scan x-ray.

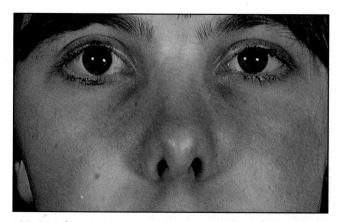

188 Otosclerosis. This is a common cause of bilateral symmetrical conductive hearing loss in adults.

The stapes footplate is ankylosed in the <u>oval</u> window by thick vascular bone. This curious bony lesion is usually an isolated middle-ear focus. It may be associated, however, with osteogenesis imperfecta tarda, and blue sclerae are occasionally seen with otosclerosis.

Otosclerosis is familial and more common in women (otosclerotic hearing loss increases during pregnancy, which may account for the apparently higher incidence in women). Patients frequently notice paracusis, in which there is improved hearing with background noise. The cause of otosclerosis remains unknown.

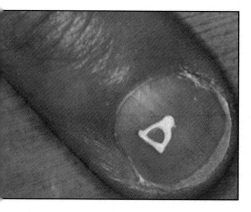

189 The stapes. The smallest bone in the body. It is, like the other ossicles, adult size at birth.

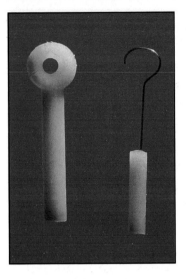

190 Stapedectomy—the prostheses. The operation for hearing loss due to otosclerosis involves removal of the ankylosed stapes bone and replacement with a mobile prosthesis. There are several types of prosthesis, of which teflon (left) and teflon-wire are the most commonly used. This very successful operation was devised by John Shea of Memphis, Tennessee, USA in 1957, and was a great advance in surgery, with good hearing achieved in over 90% of cases.

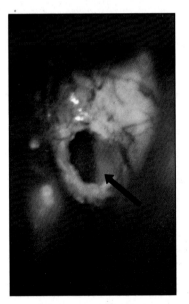

191 Stapedectomy—opening in the fixed footplate. An opening is made in the fixed footplate (shown here). The white marks to the right of this opening into the inner ear are the otoliths.

The prosthesis is attached to the long process of the incus, and the distal end of the prosthesis is placed into the inner ear.

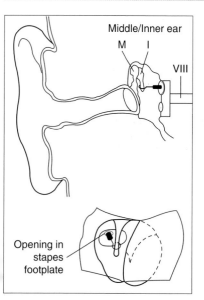

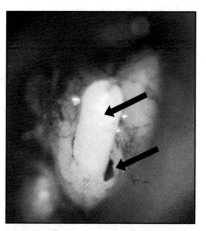

193 A teflon-wire prosthesis (*top arrow*). The distal end is entering the inner ear through the hole in the footplate (*bottom arrow*).

192 The stapedectomy operation.

The top diagram shows the attachment of the stapes prosthesis to the long process of the incus; the distal end of the prosthesis is placed through the opening made in the ankylosed stapes footplate.

The lower diagram shows the exposure of the middle ear for stapedectomy. The drum is reflected anteriorly, hinging on the long process of the malleus. The stapes superstructure and part of the footplate are removed, and the prosthesis inserted.

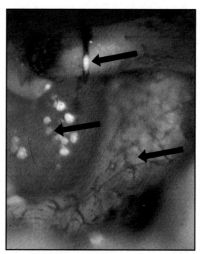

194 Teflon wire prosthesis. The wire loop is closed on the incus (*top arrow*) and a fat graft (*middle* arrow) seals the oval window. The bone covering the facial nerve (*bottom arrow*) and margin of the round window are also seen.

MICROSURGERY

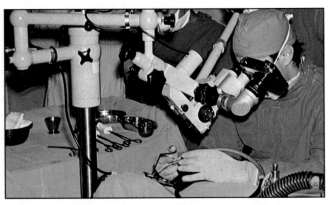

195 The middle-ear operating microscope. Middle-ear surgery is possible because of the development of the middle-ear operating microscope. This apparatus makes the drum, ossicles and other middle-ear structures easy to manipulate with fine instruments.

The microscope is either sterilised with a drape or an antiseptic, and a camera and tutor arm can be attached.

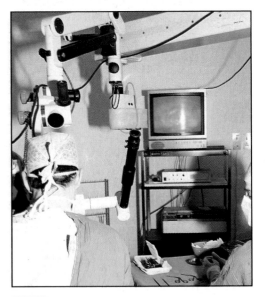

196 Operating micro-scope. A television camera can also be attached to the microscope, with a monitor giving the surgeon and observers a good operative view.

FACIAL PALSY

Facial palsy may follow skull fracture or facial nerve laceration near the stylo-mastoid foramen, and is also an uncommon complication of middle-ear surgery and superficial parotidectomy. An extensive cholesteatoma or middle-ear carcinoma may also damage the facial nerve. In the absence of a careful examination of the tympanic membrane, such a case may be wrongly diagnosed and treated as Bell's palsy. All facial palsies should have an otological assessment.

Bilateral facial palsy is an interesting rarity. It is the facial asymmetry of facial palsy that is conspicuous and makes the diagnosis obvious; a bilateral facial palsy may not be so readily diagnosed.

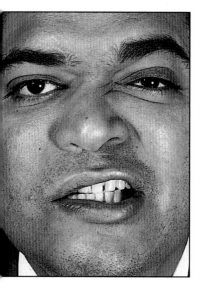

197 Bell's palsy is the commonest cause of facial palsy. It is a lower motor-neurone lesion of the facial nerve, of unknown aetiology, involving a loss of movement of facial muscles, usually total, of one side of the face. This includes the muscles of the forehead (with facial paralysis due to an upper motor-neurone lesion, such as a stroke, these muscles continue to function due to cross innervation distal to the cortex). Pain in or around the ear frequently precedes Bell's palsy, and a history of draught on the side of the face may be significant. Bell's palsy may be recurrent and associated with parotid swelling (Melkersson's syndrome).

The aetiology and management of Bell's palsy is controversial. Oedema of the facial nerve near the stylo-mastoid foramen has been demonstrated, but the cause is unknown. Most of Bell's palsies recover completely and spontaneously within six weeks. Physiotherapy maintains tone in the facial muscles during recovery, and it is probable that oral steroids (prednisolone) in high doses* in the early stage of Bell's palsy improve the prognosis.

*20 mg q.d.s. 5 days: 20 mg t.d.s. 1 day: 20 mg b.d. 1 day: 20 mg o.d. 1 day: 10 mg o.d. 1 day.

The facial nerve: tests to diagnose the level of the lesion

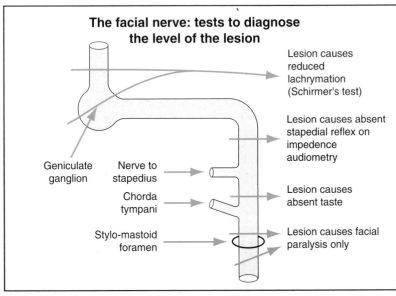

Lesion causes reduced lachrymation (Schirmer's test)

Lesion causes absent stapedial reflex on impedence audiometry

Geniculate ganglion

Nerve to stapedius

Lesion causes absent taste

Chorda tympani

Stylo-mastoid foramen

Lesion causes facial paralysis only

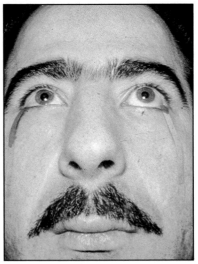

198,199 Tests of facial nerve involvement. The level of involvement of the facial nerve in facial palsy can be determined by :

1 Taste (electrogustometry, page 39): if taste is absent or impaired, the lesion is proximal to the chorda tympani.

2 Stapedial reflex (see p.18, impedance audiometry).

3 Lacrimation (Schirmer's test, **199,** left). Litmus paper is placed under the lower lid. If the facial nerve lesion is proximal to, or involves the geniculate ganglion, the tears are reduced.

These tests are reliable in traumatic section of the facial nerve to detect the level of injury. In Bell's palsy, the tests are of little value.

Chapter 3

The Nose

DEFORMITIES

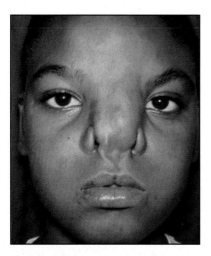

200 Congenital deformities. Abnormal fusion of the nasal processes is uncommon, and may result in varying degrees of deformity.

In this case, the nose is bifid with hypertelorism (the distance between the eyes being greatly increased). In milder cases, the bifid appearance of the nose is less marked, and may just appear as a rather 'wide' nose.

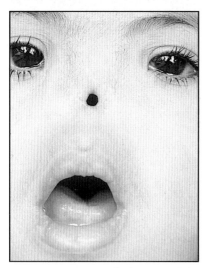

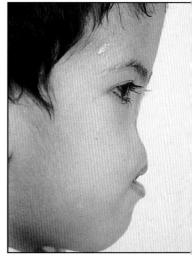

201, 202 Congenital absence of the nose is a rarity. With total atresia, this condition, as with bilateral atresia of the posterior choanae, presents an airway obstruction emergency.

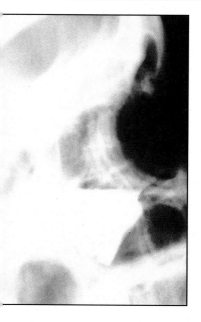

203 Congenital atresia of one posterior choana. This congenital deformity may not present until adult life. A **total unilateral obstruction** from birth may cause surprisingly little trouble to the patient. If, however, the symptoms are marked, the atresia can be treated surgically with removal of the bony obstruction. **Bilateral atresia** presents with dyspnoea soon after birth. Immediate surgical correction is required. A membranous atresia may be perforated and dilated using metal sounds, but if the atresia is bony it must be opened with a drill, using either a trans-nasal or trans-palatal approach. Indwelling portex tubes are left in place for up to 6 weeks post-operatively to prevent a recurrence of the stenosis.

Choanal atresia is well demonstrated on x-ray when an opaque medium is used to fill the nasal fossa, but a CT scan is now the diagnostic investigation used.

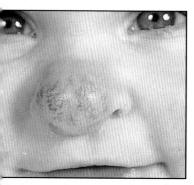

204 Haemangiomas. These are seen in children and are a cosmetic problem. Treatment is deferred, for this lesion may regress before adolescence.

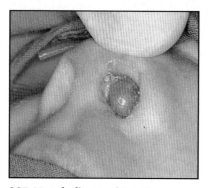

205 Nasal glioma. This curious polypoid swelling presents in the noses of children or babies. A biopsy confirms the nasal glioma, which is usually an isolated entity attached to the septum. A CT scan is needed to exclude the possibility of an intracranial attachment, but this is rare. This is a benign lesion.

CYSTS

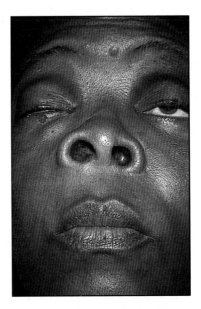

206 Naso-alveolar cysts. These are more common inBlacks, and because of their constant anatomical site, spot diagnosis is possible.

Externally, there is flattening of the naso-labial fold and flaring of the alae nasi. In the anterior nares the cyst extends into the floor of the nose and displaces the inferior turbinate upwards. Excision via a sublabial incision and enucleation is the treatment. Surgical rupture of the cyst usually means incomplete removal, and predisposes to recurrence. *Arrow* indicates 'flaring' of ala.

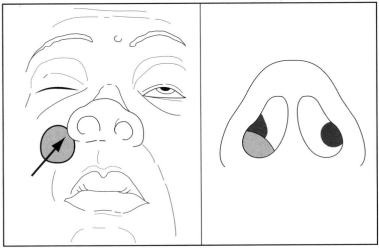

207 Naso-alveolar cysts.

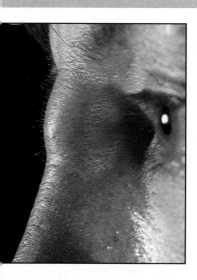

208 Dermoid. A cystic swelling near the glabella is probably a dermoid; excision may not be straightforward. The differential diagnosis in childhood is the nasal glioma.

There is commonly a sinus connecting the cyst to a punctum on the skin near the nasal tip, and there may be extension of the cyst deep to the nasal bones as far as the cribriform plate.

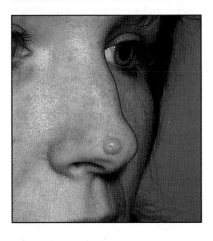

209 Nasal papilloma. Benign lesions on the nose such as a mole or papilloma are common. If large, however, the obvious site on the nose necessitates excision and biopsy.

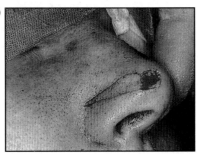

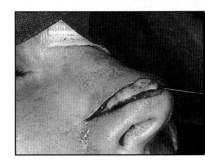

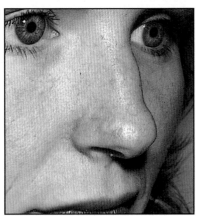

210–212 Nasal papilloma excision. Excision is not straightforward. An elliptical excision (**210**) with closure (**211**) will produce an obvious nasal asymmetry (**212**), and more elaborate techniques are required to ensure a satisfactory result.

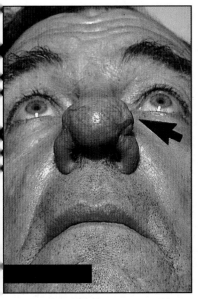 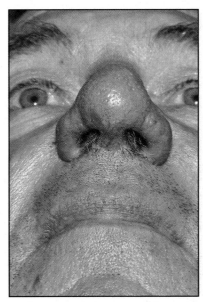

213, 214 Rhinophyma, in which the skin becomes thickened and vascular, may produce gross nasal deformity in which the skin epithe-lium becomes grossly thickened and vascular. 'Shaving' of the excess skin (without skin grafting) is the surgical treatment. Irregular areas of epithelium (*arrow*) should be sent for histology since **basal- or squamous-cell carcinoma** may occur within a rhinophyma.

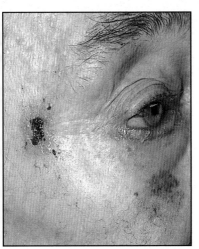

215 Basal-cell carcinoma (rodent-cell carcinoma) are common on the nose, face and ear. Any persistent ulcer, which may bleed, or area of induration should arouse suspicion. Excision or radio-therapy is curative for early lesions. Deeply erosive basal-cell carcinomas may be difficult to resect or cure.

ADENOIDS

Persistent snoring is the main symptom of enlarged adenoids. Purulent rhinorrhoea (if there is secondary sinusitis) and epistaxis also occur, with or without nasal symptoms. There is hearing loss due to secretory otitis media, or earache from recurrent acute otitis media.

Adenoids normally regress before puberty and adults with large adenoids are rare. If an adult has nasal obstruction due to post-nasal lymphoid tissue, the histology is essential to exclude a lymphoma.

Nasal obstruction may occur from birth due to large adenoids, and the baby has difficulty with bottle and breast feeding. It is occasionally necessary to remove these 'congenital adenoids' in toddlers.

A conservative attitude should be taken, however, with removal of adenoids, awaiting regression of the lymphoid tissue. Adenoidectomy alone is not common surgery. Tonsillar enlargement is usually also present, and is an additional cause of the upper respiratory tract obstruction and snoring. Adenoidectomy alone is not curative, and removal of both tonsils and adenoids is necessary.

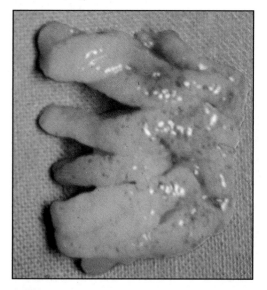

216 Adenoids. A mass of lymphoid tissue shaped like a bunch of bananas occupies the vault of the post-nasal space in children. If the adenoids are large, nasal obstruction occurs.

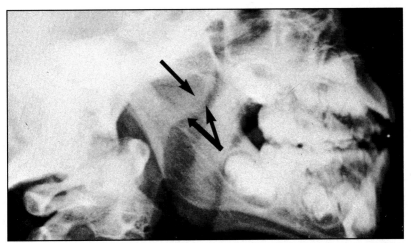

217 Lateral x-ray of adenoids. The post-nasal space is often difficult or impossible to see in a child, and a lateral x-ray clearly shows the size of the adenoids and degree of obstruction. In this x-ray, a small airway is present (*Lower arrows*) despite a large adenoid shadow (*upper arrow*).

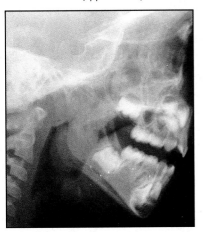
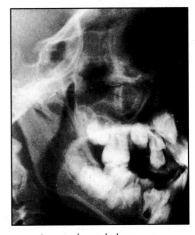

218, 219 Accurate lateral x-rays are necessary. A wrongly angled x-ray, as demonstrated here (**218**, left), is not infrequently erroneously reported as showing 'large adenoids'. It is not easy to maintain a child in the correct position; patience and skill are required by the radiographer. When checking the lateral x-ray for adenoids, therefore, it is essential to be sure that the lateral picture is true (**219**, right) before assessing the bulk of the adenoid lymphoid tissue.

TRAUMA

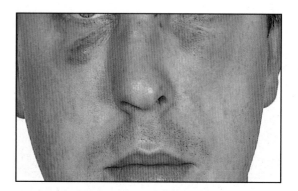

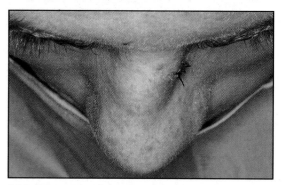

220, 221 Fractured nose. This common injury only requires treatment if the septum is dislocated or involved in haematoma, or if there is an external deviation of the nose (seen frontally as in **220** (above), and most obvious when examined from above as in **221** (below) of cosmetic concern to the patient.

It is important to reduce nasal frac-tures within two weeks, lest the bones cannot be manipulated and a subsequent rhino-plasty or re-fracture may be necessary. Reduction, therefore, is either carried out soon after the fracture or delayed until the oedema, which makes assessment of the deformity difficult, has settled (usually within 4–10 days).

Many fractured noses, however, are 'chip' or undisplaced crack fractures with haematoma, and require no treatment.

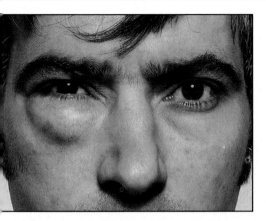

222 Surgical emphysema of the orbit. An alarming and unusual complication of a nasal fracture is surgical emphysema of the orbit when the patient blows the nose. This is due to a fracture through the ethmoidal cells and lamina papryacea, linking the nasal cavity to the orbit. There is no cause for alarm, and if care is taken not to inflate the orbit, spontaneous healing follows. The characteristic crepitus on palpation is diagnostic.

A facial injury that has caused a nasal fracture may also have involved the maxilla and anterior cranial fossa (with cerebrospinal fluid rhinorrhoea), and precautions should be taken to exclude such an associated fracture as well as any possible injury to the eye.

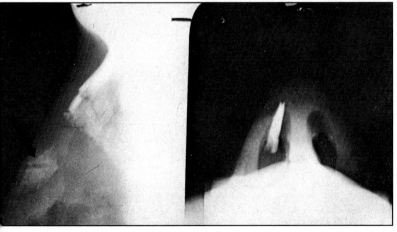

223 X-ray of nasal bones showing complete separation of one bone. In this case, the nasal bone x-ray shows some obvious and significant injury. In almost all instances, however, the x-rays for a fractured nose are of very little practical value, although they may be of medico-legal significance.

COMPLICATIONS OF A FRACTURED NOSE

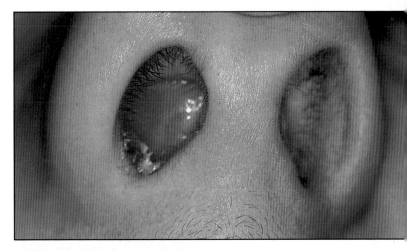

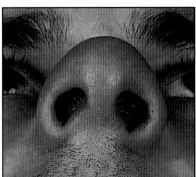
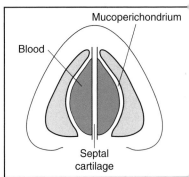

224–226 A septal haematoma following trauma to the nose. Blood collects under the subperichondrium on both sides, causing 'ballooning' of the septum and total nasal obstruction. If the nasal obstruction is ***total***, early drainage of the haematoma is required. A warning must be given pre-operatively that nasal saddling of the dorsum may ensue, the haematoma having led to necrosis of the septal cartilage. Septal swelling with partial nasal obstruction usually settles spontaneously, and drainage is not necessary.

The haematoma, if left, usually becomes infected. Pain and malaise accompany the total nasal blockage. Draining is necessary, and saddling usually inevitable (see **227** and **228**).

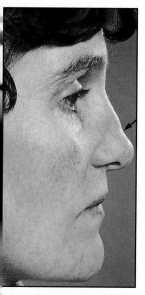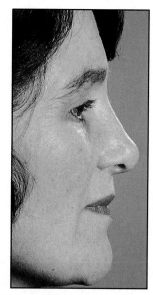

227, 228 Nasal saddling. Minimal saddling, as in this patient (**227**, left), may accentuate a previous nasal hump. Simple lowering of the nasal bones restores the appearance of a normal nose (**228**, right).

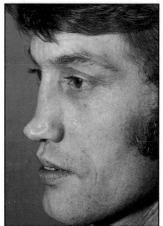

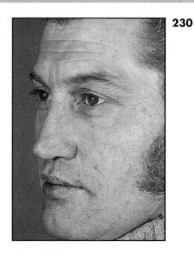

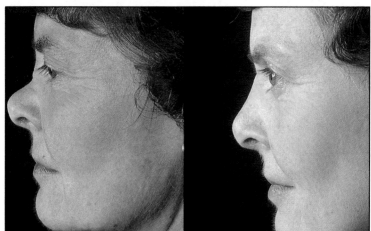

229–231 Grafts. With the more common severe saddling, a graft is needed to restore the nasal contour. Cartilage, bone or a synthetic are alternative grafting materials.

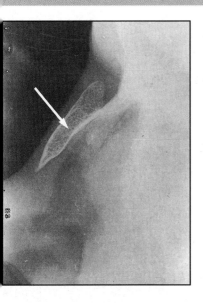

232 Iliac crest bone graft. An iliac crest bone graft (*arrow*) used for a saddle deformity is demonstrable on this x-ray.

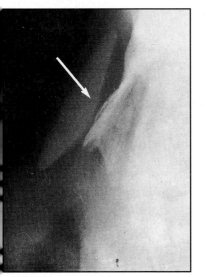

233 Synthetic graft. A synthetic graft (silastic) seen on x-ray (*arrow*), is also used to correct nasal saddling.

234–237 Septal haematomas in childhood. Septal haematomas are not uncommon in children, and may follow trauma or be spontaneous,in which case a blood dyscrasia needs to be excluded. The parents should be warned that the development of the nose may be retarded, and may ultimately lead to a 'small' nose in adult life.

In the past, surgical correction was left until the nose was fully grown at the age of 16–17 years, but it is now apparent that grafting of these saddle deformities in childhood will lead to more normal nasal development.

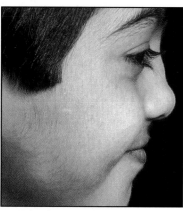

234 Before grafting (aged 7 years).

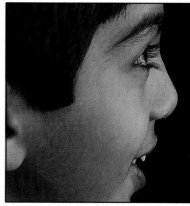

235 After grafting (aged 7 years).

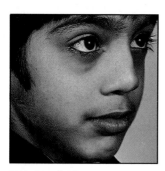

236 Aged 11 years.

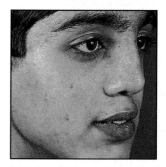

237 Aged 19 years.

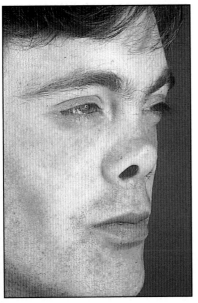 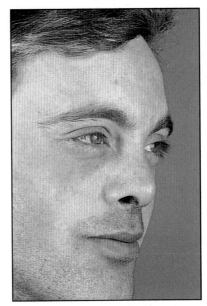

238, 239 Nasal plastic surgery using cartilage and composite ear grafts gives significant improvement to the small adult nose if saddling has resulted from a childhood septal haematoma.

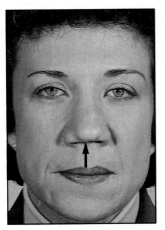

240 Retraction of the columella. Retraction of the columella and loss of tip support of the nose (arrow) are less usual complications of a septal haematoma.

241–244 Rhinoplasty. The appearance of a nose with a congenital or traumatic hump of the nasal bones can be improved with rhinoplasty (**241–244**). A deviated nose may be straightened (**245, 246**). Bulbous or bifid nasal tips can be modified (**247, 248**). Incisions for rhinoplasty are within the nasal vestibule and access to the nasal bones, cartilages, and septum is obtained with an intranasal approach.

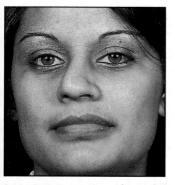
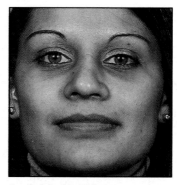

245, 246 Correction of nasal deviation with rhinoplasty.

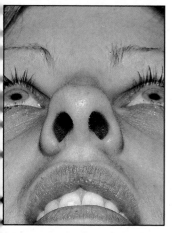
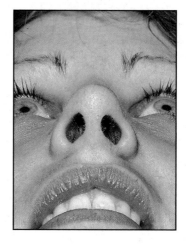

247, 248 Nasal tip rhinoplasty.

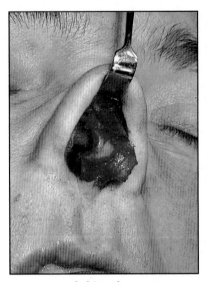 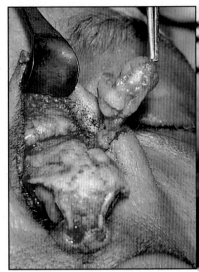

249 External rhinoplasty. A transverse incision across the columella (with a 'notch' to give a minimally perceptible scar) enables the skin of the nose to be elevated superiorly with exposure of all the underlying structures.

250 External rhinoplasty. This approach is used for many of the grosser nasal deformities, e.g. cleft-lip nasal deformities, and also enables lesions on the dorsum of the nose to be excised without an obvious overlying scar. The lesion being removed here is a nasal sinus.

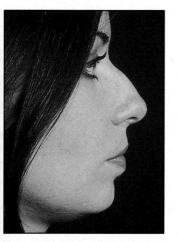
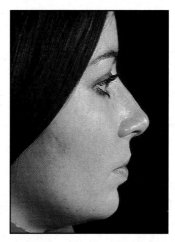

251, 252 Mentoplasty. The improvement with rhinoplasty in this case has been accentuated by mentoplasty.

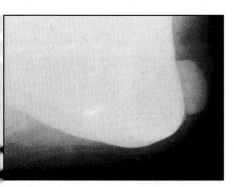

253 A silastic implant has been inserted adjacent to the mandible. A receding chin is not to be overlooked in a patient seeking rhinoplasty, for it accentuates the nasal deformity, and mentoplasty gives a subtle but striking improvement in appearance.

DEVIATED NASAL SEPTUM

A congenital or traumatic dislocation of the septal cartilage into one nasal fossa causes unilateral nasal obstruction. If the obstruction is marked, or complicated by recurrent sinusitis, a septal correction is minor and effective surgery.

The established and time-honoured operation for this is a ***submucous resection (SMR)***, but septoplasty techniques in which cartilage is preserved and repositioned—rather than removed—are now more widely used. The SMR operation involves removal of much of the septal cartilage and loss of nasal support with saddling, and septal perforations are occasional complications.

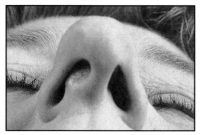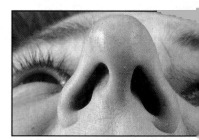

254, 255 Deviated nasal septum into the columella. With caudal dislocation of the septum, an obvious deformity is coupled with nasal obstruction. Repositioning or excision of the septal dislocation is necessary to improve the appearance and airway.

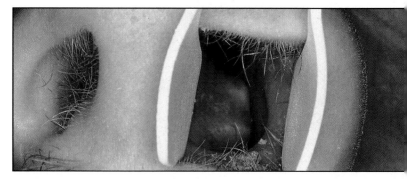

256 Deviated nasal septum. Deviated nasal septum with a spur of septal cartilage and maxillary bone occluding the inferior meatus and causing nasal obstruction.

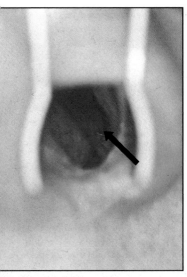

257 Septal spur indenting the inferior turbinate. A posterior deviation of the septum can be overlooked, and a vasoconstrictor applied to the anterior nasal mucous membrane reduces the size of the turbinates and allows a clear view posteriorly. *Arrow* indicates septal spur.

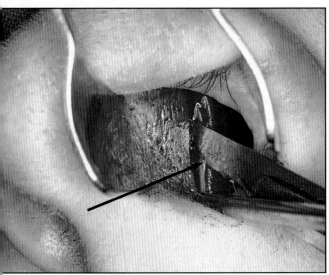

258 The septoplasty/SMR operation. An incision through the nasal mucosa and cartilage with elevation of the muco-perichondrium (*arrow*) gives access to the septal cartilage, which is partially resected and repositioned.

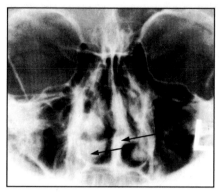

259 A posterior septal deviation. Such deviations of the vomer and ethmoid bone show on x-ray (*upper arrow*). Also seen on x-ray is the compensatory hypertrophy of the inferior turbinate on the opposite side to the deviation (*lower arrow*). It is necessary to reduce this turbinate when the septum is straightened, lest this nasal fossa becomes obstructed post-operatively.

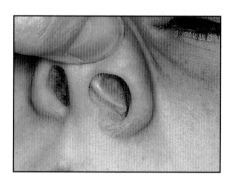

260 Deviated nasal septum in a child. The diagnosis is obvious without the use of a nasal speculum. Elevation of the infantile nasal tip suffices to give a clear view of the anterior nares.

Perforations

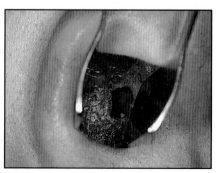

261 A perforation of the nasal septum. This may not give rise to any symptoms, and may be a chance finding on examination. Crusting usually occurs, however, causing nasal obstruction.

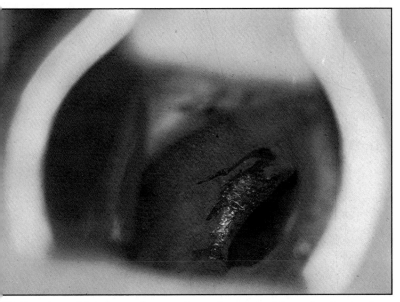

62 Prominent blood vessels appearing on the margin of the perforation, leading ⸱ epistaxis. A whistling noise on breathing is another symptom.

erforations may result from repeated trauma to the septum (e.g. nose picking); hrome workers are susceptible to a septal perichondritis causing a perforation. ⸱n inadvertent tear of the nasal mucous membrane on both sides during an SMR peration is another cause of perforation. Destruction of the vomer and ethmoid one accounts for a posterior septal perforation, and may be due to a gumma. urgical repair of septal perforations, particularly large ones, is not easy. ⸱omposite cartilage grafts taken from the concha of the ear combined with ꞑucosal rotation flaps of the nasal mucous membrane form the basis of most ⸱urrent techniques. Plastic flanged prostheses may be fitted to seal the ⸱erforation, but may extrude and may also be inhaled.

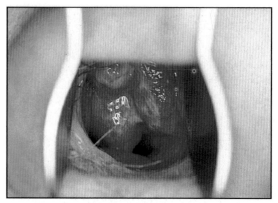

263 Granular rhinitis. Granulation tissue in the nose requires biopsy. **Sarcoidosis** not infrequently involves the upper respiratory tract mucosa of the nasal fossae and larynx. In the nose the granulations are pale, but tuberculosis, malignant granuloma and neoplasia are among the differential diagnoses.

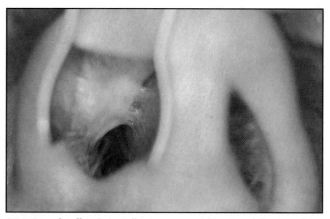

264 Nasal adhesion. Adhesions or synechiae may follow nasal trauma (including surgical trauma) and bridge the lateral wall of the nose, frequently from the inferior turbinate to the septum, causing nasal obstruction. Recurrence follows surgical division of the larger adhesions unless an indwelling silastic splint is left *in situ* until mucosa underlying the adhesion regenerates.

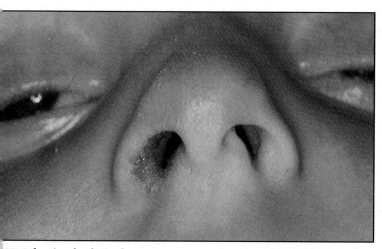

65 A foreign body in the nose causes a unilateral purulent and fetid nasal discharge. A child with these symptoms and a vestibulitis is almost certain to have a foreign body in the nose.

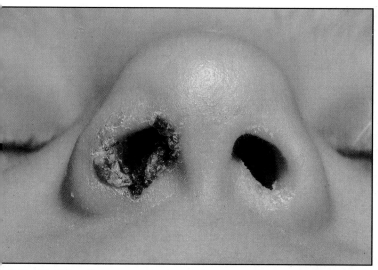

66 Vestibulitis affecting one nostril, as in this case, is almost always diagnostic of a foreign body.

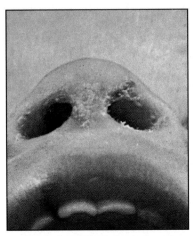

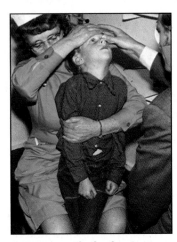

267 Vestibulitis. When nasal discharge and skin involvement affect both nostrils, a vestibulitis (an eczema of the vestibular skin) is the probable diagnosis.

268 Removal of a foreign body. Removal frequently can be managed as an outpatient, when it is necessary to hold the child securely while a probe or hook is placed posterior to the foreign body. Forceps frequently push the foreign body posteriorly, and thus should be avoided. A general anaesthetic is necessary if the foreign body is impacted or inaccessible.

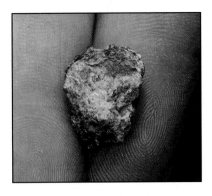

269 Rhinolith. A foreign body that is ignored accumulates a calcareous deposit and presents years later as a fetid stony hard mass—a rhinolith. This is well demonstrated on x-ray, and a rhinolith may become large eroding the lateral wall and floor of the nose. Although at first sight appearing easy to remove, the impaction may be extremely firm particularly with the larger rhinoliths.

INFLAMMATION

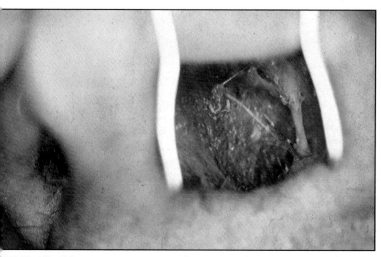

170 Vestibulitis presents as crusting and irritation in the anterior nares with result-ing nasal obstruction. Examination shows excoriated vestibular skin and septal mucous membrane. Rubbing or over-diligent cleaning of the nose by the patient usually causes vestibulitis, particularly if, as in this case, the septum is deviated anteriorly and impinges on the lateral wall of the nose. Advice and the use of anti-biotic and corticosteroid ointment are effective in controlling vestibulitis. Correction of the septum may be necessary.

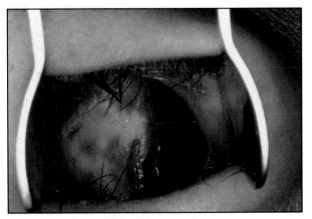

271 Nasal vestibulitis with squamous epithelium replacing the mucosa. A deviation of the septum has predisposed to a chronic vestibulitis. Digital irritation, or the use of cocaine, which may also lead to a septal perforation, may underlie this problem.

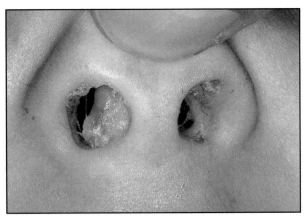

272 Vestibulitis in a child overlying a grossly deviated anterior septum. Septal surgery is avoided in children, but cases in which the obstruction is gross due to vestibulitis require a conservative septoplasty.

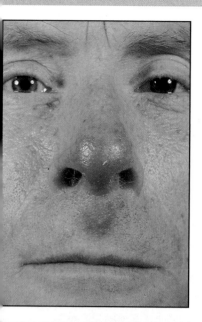

273 Furuncles and cellulitis of the columella. These may spread to involve the skin of the nose and face. Treatment is with systemic penicillin.

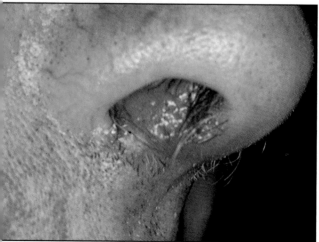

274 Furuncles and cellulitis of the columella.

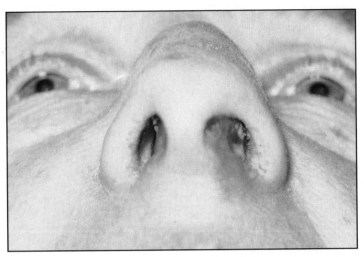

275 Vestibulitis. Painful crusting of the nasal vestibule and anterior nares may be a simple eczematous type of skin lesion which settles with a topical antibiotic and steroid. There should be, however, an awareness that this vestibulitis is a granuloma, or part of the manifestation of systemic disease such as polyarteritis nodosa or systemic lupus erythematosus. A further possibility is an 'irritative' vestibulitis from cocaine snuff, or columellar carcinoma, as in this case.

276–278 Acute rhinitis. In the common cold, the nasal mucous membrane is oedematous, so the inferior turbinate abuts against the septum to result in obstruction and an excess of mucus which causes the running nose.

A similar appearance is seen in nasal allergy, either 'seasonal hay fever' or perennial allergy, but the oedematous turbinate mucous membrane appears grey (**278**) rather than red (**277**). A persistent purulent nasal discharge usually means that there is a sinusitis. Corticosteroid nasal sprays for nasal allergy are now available, markedly reducing the obstruction, rhinorrhoea and sneezing that characterizes both seasonal and perennial nasal allergy. Skin tests to detect specific allergens are of use with grass pollen and house dust allergy related to the house dust mite.

Nasal sprays, desensitisation and oral antihistamines without sedative side-effects are the first lines of treatment for nasal allergy. This management of nasal allergy is preferable to desensitization, as there is an increased awareness and concern regarding anaphylactic shock.

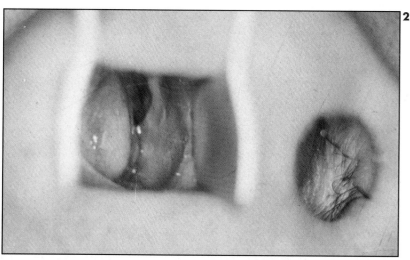

276

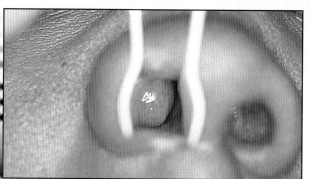

277

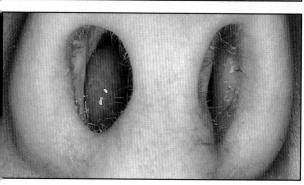

278

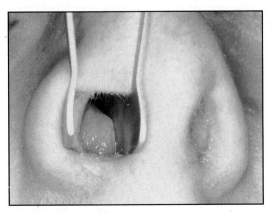

279 Chronic rhinitis. The turbinate mucous membrane frequently reacts to irritants, whether tobacco, excessive use of vasoconstrictor drops or atmospheric irritants, by enlarging. Thickened red inferior turbinates are seen adjacent to the septum, limiting the airway. Nasal obstruction, either intermittent or persistent, with a post-nasal discharge of mucus ('post-nasal drip') are the symptoms of chronic rhinitis. This is the condition most frequently labelled by the patient as 'catarrh' or 'sinus trouble'.

If the changes due to chronic rhinitis are irreversible, i.e. the nasal obstruction persists when the irritants are removed, it is probable that minor surgery to reduce the turbinates in size will be necessary. Occasionally, oral antihistamines help, but vasoconstrictor drops have no place in the treatment of chronic rhinitis, and their constant use is a common cause of this condition (*rhinitis medicamentosa*).

In most inflammatory conditions of the nasal mucous membrane, there is an excess of mucus. An atrophy of the mucosa and mucous glands with fetid crusting of wide nasal fossae, however, is seen with *atrophic rhinitis*. This is uncommon and idiopathic. It may be an isolated nasal condition, part of Wegener's granuloma or disseminated lupus erythematosus. There is also a phase of atrophic nasal crusting in rhinoscleroma.

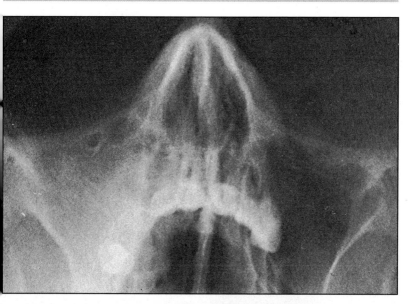

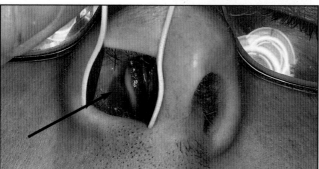

280, 281 Acute maxillary sinusitis. This is a common complication of a head cold. Apical infection of the teeth related to the antrum or an oro-antral fistula following dental extraction also cause maxillary sinusitis, as may trauma with bleeding into the antrum or barotrauma.

Frontal or facial pain may be referred to the upper teeth; nasal obstruction and purulent rhinorrhoea are the other symptoms. The antrum is opaque on x-ray (**280**, top). There may be tenderness over the sinus but swelling is rare. Pus is seen issuing from the middle meatus (**281**, bottom, *arrow*).

Acute infection may less commonly affect the ethmoid, frontal and sphenoid sinuses. Systemic antibiotics, a vasoconstrictor spray or drops and inhalations are usually curative for acute sinusitis. However, a persistent maxillary sinusitis requires surgery.

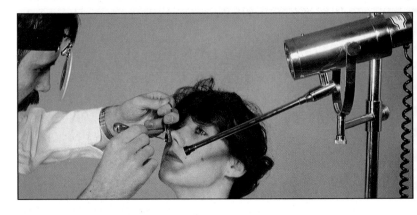

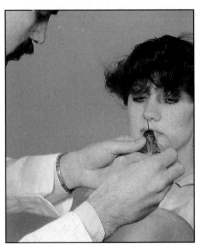

282, 283 An antral washout may be needed, albeit rarely today, for a persistent maxillary sinusitis. This involves inserting a trocar and cannula under the inferior turbinate, and puncturing the lateral wall of the nose through the maxillary process of the thin inferior turbinate bone, to enter the antrum. Water is irrigated through the cannula, and the pus emerges through the maxillary ostium. ***An acutely infected maxillary sinus must not be washed out until medical treatment has controlled the acute phase.*** Cavernous sinus thrombosis remains a danger. The bad reput-ation that antral washout has for pain is not justified if a good local anaesthetic and gentle technique are used.

Recurrent attacks of acute maxillary sinusitis may require operation. A permanent intranasal opening into the antrum is made either in the middle or inferior meatus (***intranasal antrostomy***). This operation is also effective for those cases of acute sinusitis that fail to respond to conservative treatment and antral washouts.

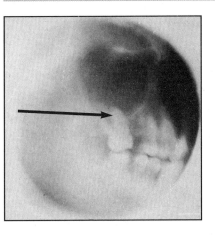

284 Dental sinusitis. The apices of the molar teeth may be extremely close to the antral mucosal lining. The upper wisdom tooth apparent on this x-ray (*arrow*), if infected, would be likely to cause maxillary sinusitis or, if removed, would be clearly at risk for causing an oro-antral fistula.

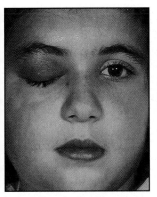

285 Orbital cellulitis. Complications of acute sinusitis con-fined to the antrum are rare. A severe maxillary sinusitis, however, usually involves the ethmoid and frontal sinuses. Infection spreading via the lamina papyracea or floor of the frontal sinus leads to an orbital cellulitis. A CT scan is essential in these cases to define the extent of infection and to exclude frontal lobe involvement.

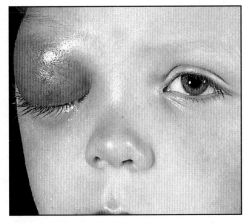

286 An orbital abscess requiring external drainage may form. Meningitis or brain abscess may also follow the spread of infection from the roof of the ethmoid, frontal or sphenoid sinus to the anterior cranial fossa. Infection associated with a rapidly growing neoplasm, such as a rhabdomyo-sarcoma, is the differential diagnosis in this case.

Chronic sinusitis

Chronic sinusitis may develop from incomplete resolution of an acute infection. The onset, however, may be insidious and secondary to nasal obstruction (e.g. due to a deviated septum, nasal polyps or, in children, to enlarged adenoids). Apical infection of the teeth related to the antra can also cause chronic sinusitis.

Purulent rhinorrhoea, nasal obstruction and headache are the main symptoms of chronic sinusitis. Pus in the middle meatus with opacity of the sinus are confirmatory of infection. Pus confined to the antrum rarely gives complications, but often there is spread of infection to the ethmoids and frontal sinuses. It is not common for frontal and ethmoidal sinusitis to occur without maxillary sinusitis. Pus in the frontal and ethmoid sinus, as with acute infections, may spread to involve the orbit and brain. Obstruction of the sinus ostium may lead to an encysted collection of mucus within the sinus—a mucocele.

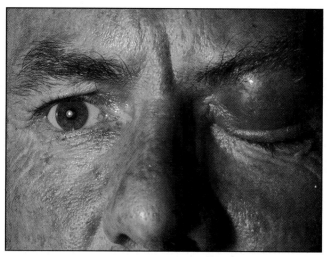

287 A mucocele. The frontal sinus is commonly affected, and erosion of the roof of the orbit leads to orbital displacement downwards and laterally.

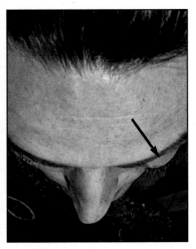

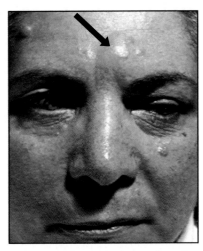

288, 289 A mucocele. Proptosis also occurs with mucoceles, and is best confirmed by examination from above (**288**, left,*arrow*). The frontal sinus wall may be eroded both posteriorly and anteriorly. An eroded anterior wall results in a fluctuant swelling on the forehead (**289**, right, *arrow*). In this case, there is also orbital displacement and proptosis.

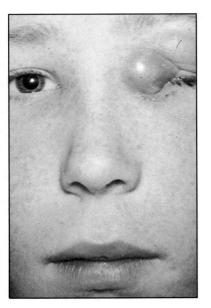

290 Lateral displacement of the orbit. This occurs with a mucocele arising in the ethmoid sinus, and is usually accompanied by a swelling at the medial canthus. In this case, the mucocele is infected—a pyocele.

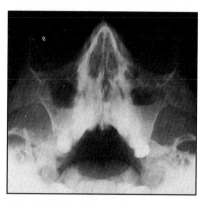
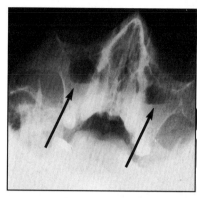

291, 292 Maxillary sinus x-rays. In acute and chronic maxillary sinusitis, a fluid level may be seen on x-ray. A tilted view is taken to confirm the presence of fluid (right, *arrows*). A thickened or rather 'straight' mucous membrane may look like a fluid level, as may a bony shadow if the x-ray is wrongly angled.

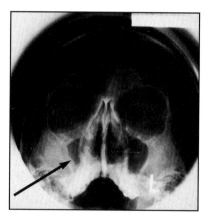
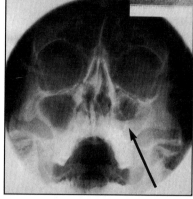

293, 294 Mucosal thickening of the antral mucosa (*arrow*) is a common finding on x-ray, indicating past sinusitis. As a 'chance' x-ray finding in the absence of other nasal symptoms or signs, it is usually not significant.

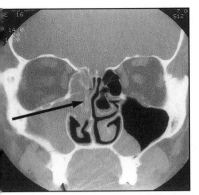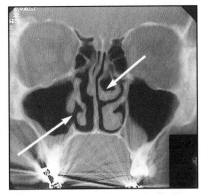

295, 296 CT scans to show the sinuses. CT scans give a much more detailed picture of the maxillary, ethmoid, frontal and sphenoid sinuses. They are routine when endoscopic sinus surgery is anticipated, and are also of additional help to the plain sinus x-rays for diagnosis. CT scans, however, involve considerably more radiation to the orbit and are expensive.

Opacity of the ethmoid sinuses characteristic of infection is seen (**295**, left, *arrow*). Also seen is an air cell in the middle turbinate (concha bullosa – **296**, right, *upper arrow*) and a right intranasal antrostomy into the maxillary sinus (*lower arrow*).

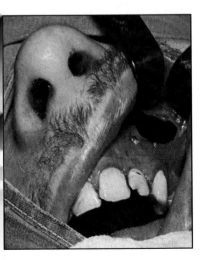

297 The Caldwell–Luc operation. Chronic maxillary sinusitis may require the Caldwell–Luc operation in which the antrum is opened with a sublabial antrostomy, the antral mucous membrane removed, and an intranasal antrostomy made. The Caldwell–Luc operation, previously very commonly carried out, is now almost a rarity. Antibiotics, endoscopic sinus surgery and a possible change in the nature of the sinus disease account for this.

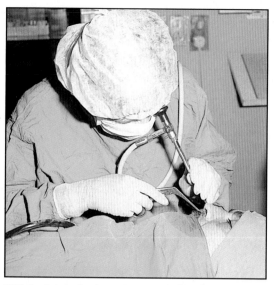

298 Endoscopic sinus surgery to the ethmoid sinuses also now helps to resolve chronicmaxillary sinusitis, and has displaced the necessity for the Caldwell–Luc operation.

Chronic frontal sinusitis may also require surgery, and is treated with an endoscopic or external approach. Obliteration of the sinus with a fat graft or enlarging the fronto-nasal duct are the two current operations.

The improvement of instruments and techniques for sinus endoscopy (see **61**) has increased the possibilities of sinus surgery. Biopsy of antral mucosa, excision of cysts and removal of foreign bodies (e.g. a misplaced apical dental filling) can be carried out via the sinus endoscope.

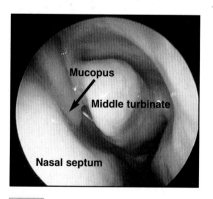

299 View through the sinus endoscope.

POLYPS

Nasal polyps are a common cause of nasal obstruction, and may cause anosmia. They are benign and do not present with bleeding. Examination shows a grey pendulous *opalescent* swelling arising from the ethmoid. A polyp is very different in appearance from the red inferior turbinate adjacent to it.

Polyps may be solitary or multiple, often extending from the nasal vestibule to the posterior choana. They are usually bilateral. Nasal polyps may become extremely large, causing expansion of the nasal bones and alae nasi. A nasal polyp which is ulcerated and bleeds is probably malignant.

Nasal polyps result from a distension of an area of nasal mucous membrane with intercellular fluid. They are due to a hypersensitivity reaction in the mucous membrane, but may also result from sinus infection. Obstruction of the sinuses by polyps, however, may lead to a secondary sinusitis, and a sinus x-ray is a routine investigation.

Small nasal polyps may cause little in the way of symptoms and may be chance findings. Usually, however, polyps extend and enlarge, and present with nasal obstruction. They do regress with corticosteroid nose drops and sprays, but in many instances, surgical removal either under local or general anaesthesia is necessary.

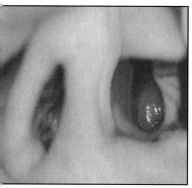

300 Nasal polyp.

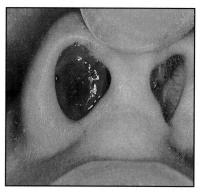

301 Nasal polyp extruding through the anterior nares. Large nasal polyps prolapse into the nasal vestibule with the exposed surface losing the opalescent grey colour.

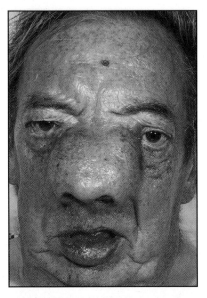

302 Extensive nasal polyps may expand into the nasal bones, and the external deformity of the polyps may become gross. Surgical removal of the polyps may suffice in the elderly in whom this complication is usually seen.

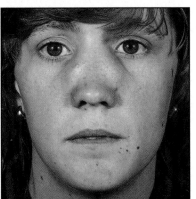 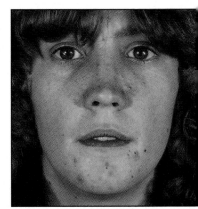

303, 304 Nasal bone expansion due to extensive nasal polypi in the younger patient also requires rhinoplasty to restore appearance.

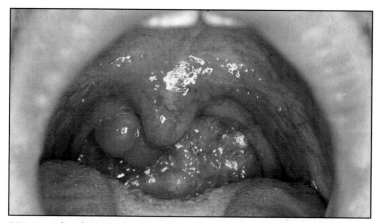

305 Nasal polyps in the oropharynx. Extensive nasal polyps may extend beyond the soft palate and present in the oropharynx.

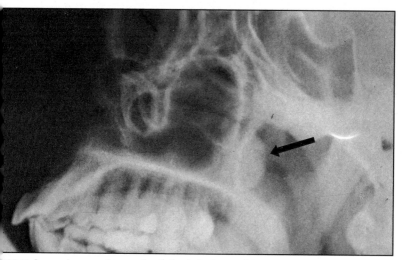

306 Enlarged posterior ends of the inferior turbinates. Turbinates may enlarge in chronic rhinitis (and in nasal allergy) to produce a large polypoid mass obstructing the posterior choanae (*arrowed*). If these cannot be seen with the post-nasal mirror, they are demonstrated on the lateral x-ray.

Antrochoanal polyp

This is a special type of nasal polyp occurring in adolescents and young adults. Unilateral nasal obstruction is caused by a grey single polyp seen in the post-nasal space. The maxillary sinus is opaque on x-ray.

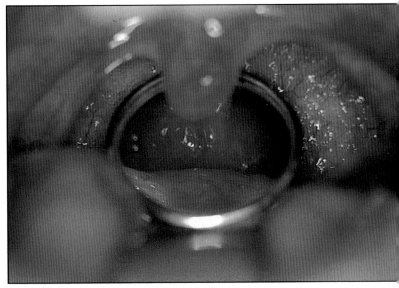

307 Antrochoanal polyp. A large antrochoanal polyp presents below the soft palate and extends into the oropharynx. A solitary polyp in one choana is almost certainly an antrochoanal polyp, but a rare vascular polyp that should be remembered as a differential diagnosis is the ***angiofibroma of male puberty***.

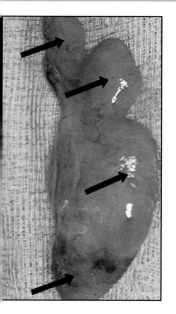

308 Antrochoanal polyp. This type of polyp, which arises from the antral mucosa, extrudes through the ostium to fill the posterior nasal fossa and post-nasal space. It frequently becomes extremely large and extends below the soft palate. Removal of the polyp from its origin in the antrum through a sublabial antrostomy approach may be necessary.

The polyp is dumb-belled in shape with a pedicle connecting the nasal and antral portions. Intranasal removal is followed by recurrence in 50% of cases, but may be necessary in early adolescence if the permanent dentition is endangered by a sublabial antrostomy. *Top arrow* shows polyp removed from antrum; *second arrow* shows polyp from nasal fossa; *third arrow* indicates polyp from post-nasal space; *bottom arrow* indicates polyp that has extended into oropharynx.

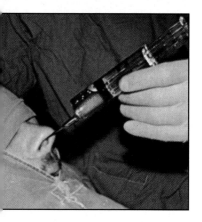

309 Aspiration from the antrum. This shows straw–coloured fluid, and is a reliable diagnostic test for an antrochoanal polyp.

EPISTAXIS

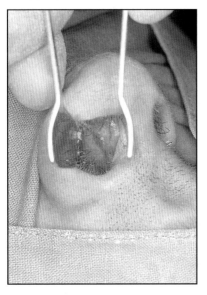

310 Epistaxis. Anteriorly on the septum there is anastomosis of several arteries (the sphenopalatine, the greater palatine, the superior labial and the anterior ethmoidal). This site is called Little's area or Kiesselbach's plexus, and is the commonest site of nose bleeds.

Although associated with alarm, most epistaxis is short-lived and trivial. It is better to sit upright since the blood tends to be swallowed, causing nausea on lying down.

There are numerous causes of epistaxis. Some, such as trauma and acute inflammatory nasal conditions, are obvious and common, but the more serious local and general causes must not be overlooked. Diagnosis must follow control of the epistaxis. Hypertension and blood dyscrasia are important general causes; neoplasms and telangiectasia may also be underlying local factors.

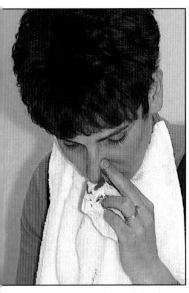

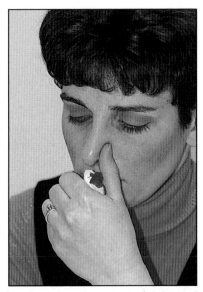

311, 312 Control of epistaxis. Firm pressure with the finger or thumb on the lateral wall of the nose opposite Little's area on the side of the bleeding, if maintained for about four minutes, will control the bleeding.

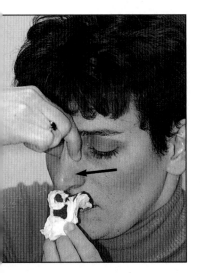

313 Incorrect technique for controlling epistaxis. The pressure is over the nasal bones and ineffective. *Arrow* indicates site where pressure should be applied.

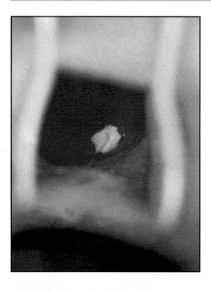

314 Cautery. If epistaxis is recurrent, cautery (which is painless with local anaesthetic) to the bleeding point is necessary, either with galvano-cautery or with a chemical (e.g. trichloracetic acid o silver nitrate). Trichloracetic acid used in this case causes the bleeding site in Little's area to become white.

Care must be taken to avoid the chemicals running onto the skin of the vestibule or face, as scarring will result. A topical anaesthetic is applied to the nasal mucous membrane in Little's area for galvano-cautery but, with silver nitrate and trichloracetic acid, no anaesthetic is needed, and the procedure is painless providing the vestibular skin is not touched.

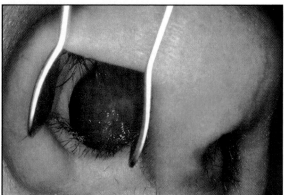

315 Hereditary nasal telangiectasia. Frequent and often severe epistaxis is characteristic of this condition, in which numerous leashes of bleeding vessels are apparent over Little's area of the nasal septum (and to be seen elsewhere, e.g. in the hands or over the trunk).

Cautery may be effective in the early stages, but this condition is difficult to manage, and may require either extensive skin grafting of the nasal septum to replace the vascula septal mucosa or oestrogen therapy.

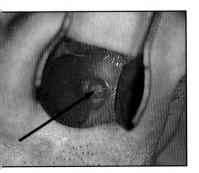

316 Septal hemangioma. A vascular sessile polyp is seen on the septum (haemangioma), which is the cause of severe, recurrent bleeds. Treatment is by excision, or cautery if the lesion is small.

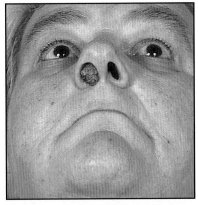

317 A large septal hemangioma occluding the nasal vestibule. Sometimes this is called a "bleeding polypus of the septum".

Epistaxis from the anterior septum may be profuse and alarming, but firm sustained pressure on the nares is invariably effective. Posterior epistaxis from the sphenopalatine artery may be very severe and difficult to manage. Nasal packing is needed to control the acute phase, and ligation of the maxillary or external carotid artery is necessary if bleeding is persistent or severe.

The terminal branch of the anterior ethmoidal artery may be the site of bleeding superiorly in the nose, particularly with nasal fractures; this vessel may require ligation. Radiographic techniques enable embolism of the terminal vessels to be carried out via an arterial catheter, and this is an option in managing very severe epistaxis, which may become life-threatening.

NEOPLASMS

MALIGNANT NASAL TUMOURS

A nasal polyp that does not appear grey and opalescent should arouse suspicion as should a polyp that bleeds spontaneously. A solid-looking hyperaemic polyp may be an ***inverted papilloma***. Granulation tissue in the nose may be malignant granuloma or carcinoma, and biopsy of any suspicious nasal lesion is necessary.

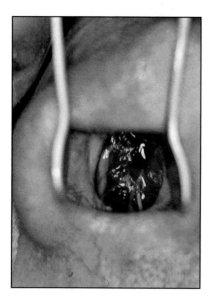

318 A pigmented polyp may be a malignant melanoma.

Prognosis when radiotherapy is followed by maxillectomy is quite good for an early maxillary carcinoma, but poor when there is extensive invasion. Exenteration of the orbit with maxillectomy is necessary when the base of the skull is inoperable. The use of cytotoxic drugs results in regression in some of these paranasal sinus neoplasms and is a further line of treatment. Extension of neoplasm superiorly into the anterior cranial fossa involves resection superiorly of the dura and involved frontal lobe of the brain in continuity with the nasal and sinus neoplasms (cranio-facial resection).

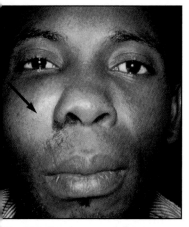

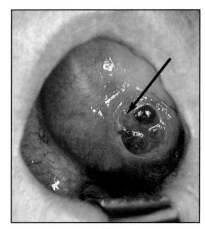

19, 320 Carcinoma of the antrum or ethmoid. These may extend not only into the nasal fossa and cheek (**319,** left, *arrow*), but may present in the oral cavity (**320, ꜱꜱʜt,** *arrow*), appearing as a dental lesion.

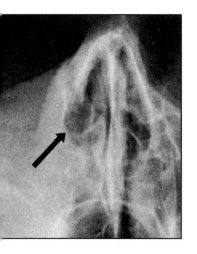

321 X-ray of antrum. The antrum is opaque on x-ray, and a CT scan will show evidence of bony destruction (*arrowed*) .

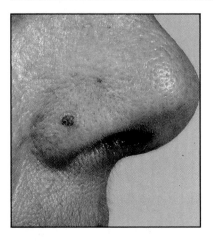

322 Basal-cell carcinoma of the nose. One should be suspicious of an apparently innocent but chronic skin lesion (*arrow*) which slowly increases in size and may bleed. Excision with a good margin is curative. If, however, these lesions are ignored—and frequently they are disguised with cosmetics for months and even years—their excision can present considerable problems of re-construction to avoid deformity in such an obvious site as the region of the nasal tip

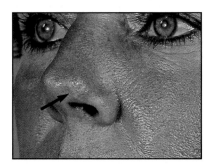

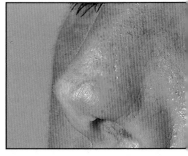

323, 324 Repair following excision of nasal tip basal-cell carcinoma. A large defect may remain in an obvious site (*arrow*). In this instance, a composite graft (graft of two or three tissue layers) taken from the cartilage and skin of the ear was used as a free graft to repair the nasal tip.

Basal-cell carcinomas in the groove at the base of the alae tend to erode deeply. Radiotherapy is the alternative treatment to surgery, and with modern super-voltage therapy, lesions overlying cartilages can be treated with minimal risk of perichondritis.

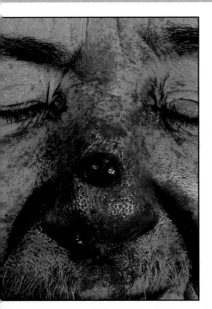

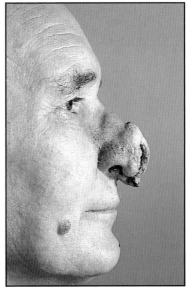

325 Carcinoma of the nose. The apex of the nasal vestibule must be examined extremely carefully in a case of scanty epistaxis, where no obvious bleeding site is apparent.

Minimal bleeding and occasional serosanguineous discharge were this patient's presenting complaints.

Later, the carcinoma became obvious, having eroded through the skin of the dorsum of the nose. Treatment with radiotherapy in this case was curative. Wide surgical excision with reconstruction of the nose was the alternative treatment.

326 Carcinoma of the nose. Wide surgical excision with forehead reconstruction rhinoplasty or, less commonly, radiotherapy, are the available treatments.

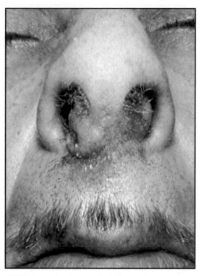

327 Carcinoma of the septum and columella.

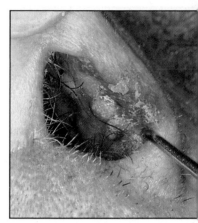

328 Squamous-cell carcinoma of the nasal vestibule. The history was short, and the differential diagnosis of a basal-cell carcinoma was made at biopsy.

329 Carcinoma of the nasal septum. A biopsy of this ulcer on the septum and columella which presented with scanty epistaxis confirmed squamous-cell carcinoma.

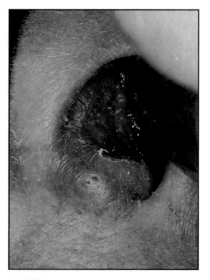

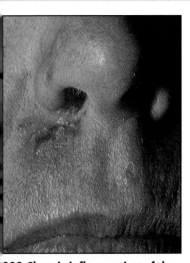

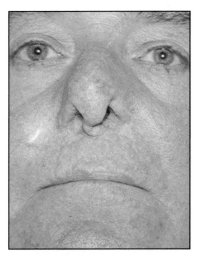

330 Chronic inflammation of the nose. *Lupus vulgaris* is now rare. It presents as a chronic ulcer of the nasal vestibule extending on to the face. The differential diagnosis of inflammatory ulceration anteriorly in the nose includes sarcoidosis, which may also cause destruction of the ala. Biopsy is necessary for the diagnosis.

331 The effects of lupus vulgaris. Lupus, if ignored, is destructive to the skin and cartilage of the alae nasi and septum.

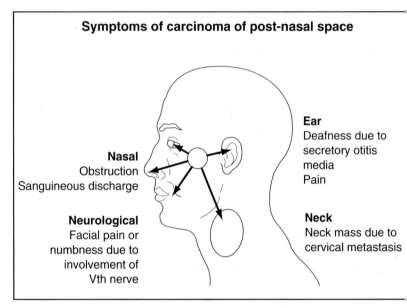

Symptoms of carcinoma of post-nasal space

Nasal
Obstruction
Sanguineous discharge

Ear
Deafness due to
secretory otitis
media
Pain

Neurological
Facial pain or
numbness due to
involvement of
Vth nerve

Neck
Neck mass due to
cervical metastasis

332 Carcinoma of the post-nasal space (nasopharynx). This is uncommon in most countries, but has an unexplained high incidence in the Far East (particularly China) and East Africa.

There are many presenting symptoms. As the posterior choanae are large, nasal obstruction is not common with ulcerated carcinomas, which tend to present with symptoms of nerve involvement or secretory otitis media due to interference with the Eustachian tube. Lymphosarcomas and papilliferous carcinomas, however, cause obstruction. Carcinoma invades the skull base involving the Vth, VIth and Vidian (pterygoid) nerves, and may cause headache by invasion of the dura. The nasopharynx is a relatively concealed site, and presentation of carcinoma is commonly late, with a cervical node metastasis.

The treatment is with radiotherapy. The overall prognosis is not good, with about a 30% five-year survival rate. This is, however, mainly related to the late diagnosis. An awareness of the early presenting symptoms and signs is essential for improved prognosis.

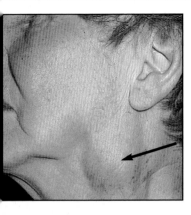

333 Carcinoma of the post-nasal space, presenting with a metastatic cervical lymph node (*arrow*).

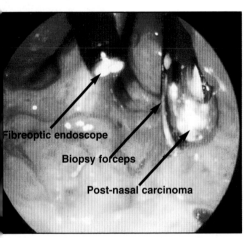

Fibreoptic endoscope

Biopsy forceps

Post-nasal carcinoma

334 Carcinoma of the post-nasal space. A photograph through the fibreoptic endoscope gives a clear view of this post-nasal space carcinoma.

The biopsy forceps also introduced through the anterior nares can be seen. Biopsy therefore of a post-nasal carcinoma can be carried out as an outpatient procedure under local anaesthetic, using the fibreoptic endoscope.

Prior to the introduction of this instrument, the post-nasal space was a 'hidden' site, as this area cannot always be seen with mirror examination (see **53**). General anaesthesia was necessary for a thorough examination and biopsy.

01223 884 825

01223 885 893

Chapter 4

The Pharynx and Larynx

THE OROPHARYNX, MOUTH AND LIPS

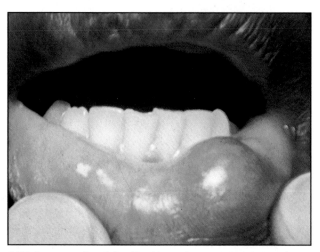

335 A mucocele of the lip. Mucoceles are cystic, non-tender swellings presenting on the lips or in the oral cavity. They result from extravasation of mucus from a mucous gland into the surrounding tissue. Treatment is excision, which is not always easy because of the extremely thin wall. Simple marsupialisation is often adequate.

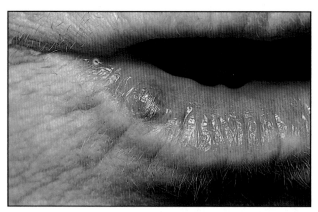

336 A haemangioma of the lip. These may require excision or laser surgery from a cosmetic point of view or on account of bleeding with trauma.

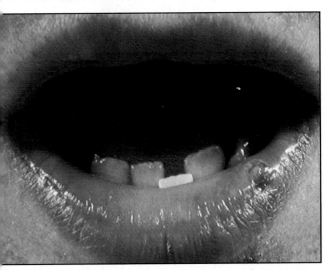

337 Lip ulcers. Lip ulceration has numerous causes, either traumatic, inflammatory or neoplastic. The provisional diagnosis can be made from the history and type of ulcer. Biopsy is necessary to confirm the diagnosis.

This lesion is a ***pyogenic granuloma***. Although these lesions are frequently small and related to trauma, they may enlarge from secondary infection (see **338**) and take several weeks to heal.

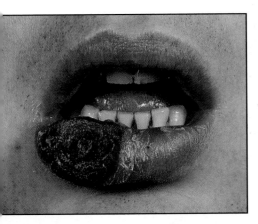

338 Lip ulcer enlarging from secondary infection.

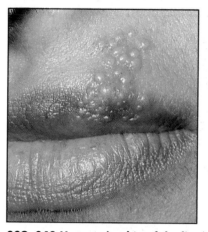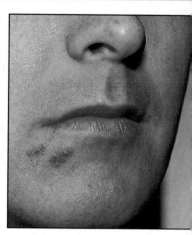

339, 340 Herpes simplex of the lip showing the characteristic vesicles (**339**, left) which later crust (**340**, right).

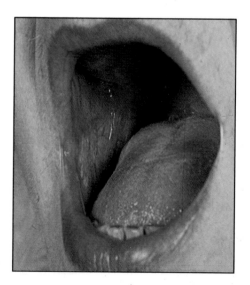

341 Keratosis may extend from the angle of the mouth along the occlusal plane of the teeth, and is commonly a dental problem; it may be self-induced due to nervous cheek-biting. It is often the result of persistent trauma to the mucous membrane.

When occurring in a site not exposed to trauma, e.g. the retro-molar fossa, it should arouse suspicion that the mucosal change may be malignant and therefore a biopsy is necessary.

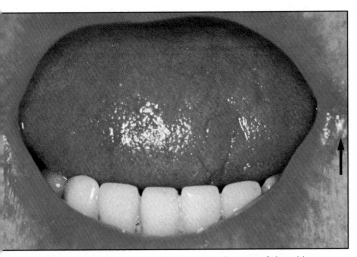

342 Angular stomatitis (*arrowed*) occurs with the type of dental hyper-keratosis shown in **341**, but it may also be part of the Plummer–Vinson or Patterson–Brown–Kelly syndromes in which glossitis (also seen here) and hypochromic anaemia are associated with a post-cricoid lesion, either a web or a carcinoma. This syndrome occurs mostly in women.

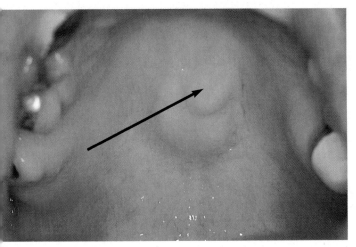

343 The torus palatinus. The bony hard mid-line palatal swelling can be diagnosed confidently by these characteristics (*arrow*). It is a common finding, and only requires removal if it interferes with the fitting of a denture.

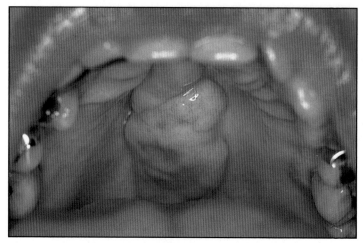

344 A large torus palatinus may take on a curious, irregular appearance suspicious of a carcinoma. Similar bony swellings occur on the lingual surface of the lower alveolus opposite the pre-molars (torus mandibularis).

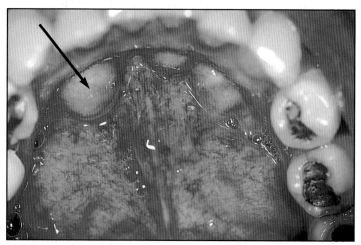

345 Torus mandibularis. A white bony hard lesion arising from the inner aspect of the mandible may present as a swelling in the floor of the mouth (*arrow*). This is considerably less common than the torus palatinus.

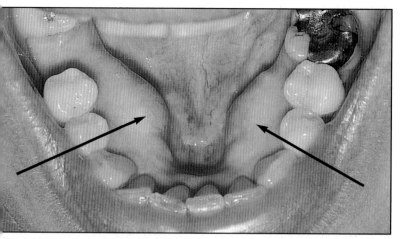

46 A bilateral torus mandibularis (*arrows*).

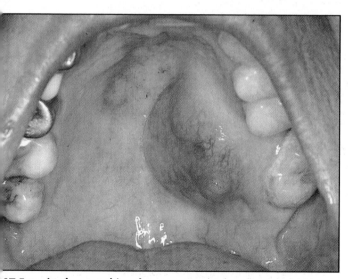

47 Ectopic pleomorphic adenoma. A palatal swelling which is not bony and hard may be a fissural cyst if mid-line, but if placed to one side (as here), it is almost certainly a tumour of one of the minor salivary glands. Biopsy is necessary. It is frequently a pleomorphic adenoma, but may be an adenoid cystic carcinoma or other malignant salivary tumour. A tumour extension from the maxillary antrum must also be excluded.

APTHOUS ULCERS

An area of white superficial ulceration is surrounded by a hyperaemic mucous membrane. These commonly occur in crops of two or more, and heal spontaneously in about one week. They are also acutely tender, and affect the non keratinised oral mucous membrane. Although there is no induration on palpation, the histological inflammatory changes are not superficial, and may extend into the underlying muscle.

Hydrocortisone pellets to suck, or triamcinolone with Orabase ointment applied to the ulcer, are the most effective present treatments to relieve the pain. As the aetiology of these extremely common ulcers remains unknown, treatment is empirical.

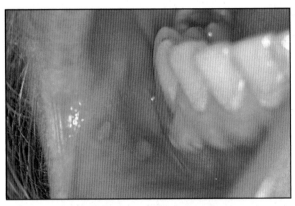

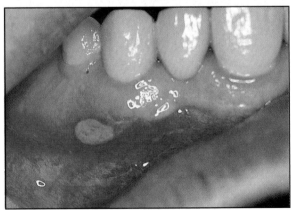

348, 349 Aphthous ulcers.

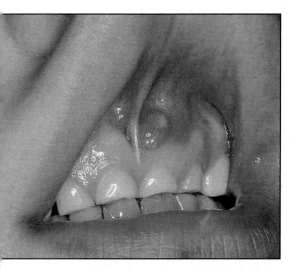

350 Ulceration and swelling of dental origin. An aphthous-like ulcer overlying the apex of this deciduous tooth suggests the diagnosis of an apical dental abscess.

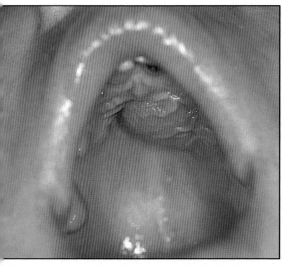

351 Ulceration and swelling of dental origin.

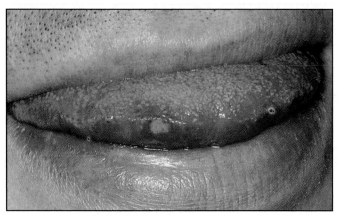

352 Apthous ulcers on the tongue. Aphthous ulcers on the tongue margin are often traumatic from tooth irregularity.

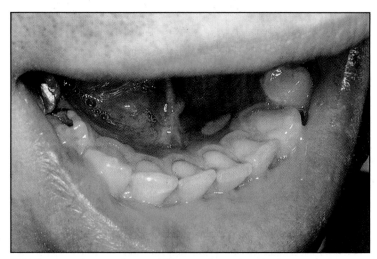

353 Trauma from a denture. This may be an irritating factor, as may any minor trauma to the mucous membrane in a person susceptible to aphthous ulcers.

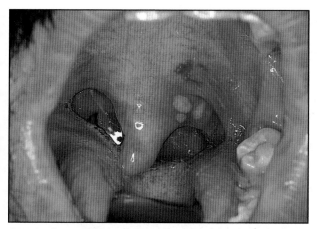

354 Apthous ulcers on the soft palate. Aphthous ulcers are
not uncommon on the soft palate.

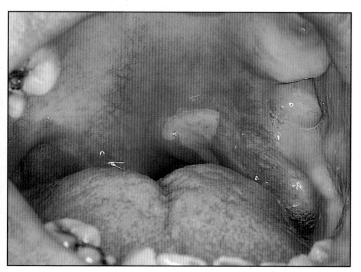

355 Solitary aphthous ulcer. This ulcer (***periadenitis mucosa
necrotica recurrens***) looks similar to a simple aphthous ulcer and is the
same histologic-ally, but it behaves differently. It is less common, larger, persists for several weeks or months and may leave a scar. It occurs in more
varied sites affect-ing the soft palate and even the pyriform fossa, where it
presents with severe dysphagia. Carbenoxolone is used topically for the
lesions in the oral cavity.

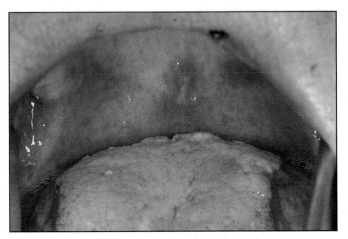

356 Multiple oral ulcers. These may be the herpetiform type of aphthous ulceration, but are possibly caused by a blood dyscrasia. If the ulcers are crusted and haemorrhagic, the condition is either erythema multiforme or pemphigus. An iritis and genital ulceration may be present (Behçets syndrome).

High doses of systemic steroids are usually needed to control this type of severe ulceration. The snail-track ulcers of secondary syphilis must be remembered also in the differential diagnosis of oral ulceration (see **410**).

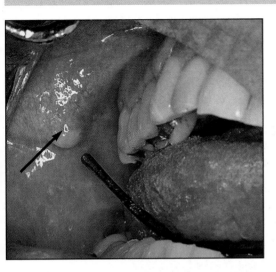

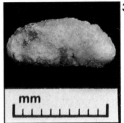

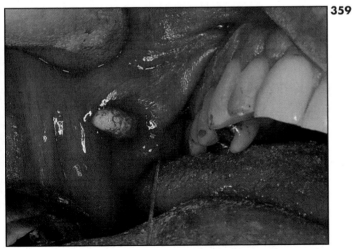

357–359 Parotid salivary calculus. An ulcer in the region of the orifice of the parotid duct (**357**, *arrow*) suggests a possible salivary calculus. Parotid calculi are considerably less common than those in the sub-mandibular duct, but occasionally they may occlude the orifice of the duct, causing painful intermittent parotid swelling which requires incision and removal (**358** and **359**).

THE TONGUE

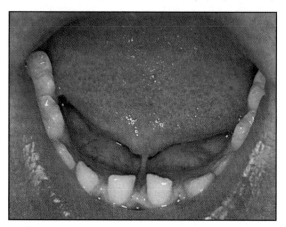

360 'Tongue tie'. This is due to a short frenulum linguae, and apart from the defect of being unable to protrude the tongue, the patient is almost always symptom-free. Speech defects can rarely be attributed to tongue-tie necessitating division of the frenulum. Division is carried out under general anaesthetic, and a suture may be required.

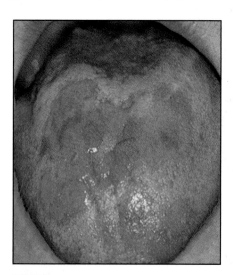

361 Geographic tongue (benign migratory glossitis). There are smooth areas with no filiform papillae. These areas vary in site on the tongue, and the appearance may concern the patient. It is, however, a condition of no significance requiring no treatment other than reassurance.

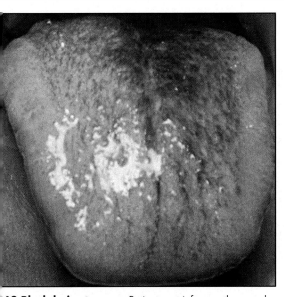

362 Black hairy tongue. Patients not infrequently regard ʈe appearance of their tongue as an index of their general ʰealth, and are concerned upon seeing a brown-black ʳaining. This may be fungal (*Aspergillus niger*) and related to ʳrolonged antibiotic therapy, but is frequently a chance finding ʷith no other pathology than hypertrophy of the filiform ᵖapillae. Tobacco may be a cause. Scraping and cleaning the ᵒngue temporarily improves the appearance, but is unneces-ᵃry since this condition is harmless.

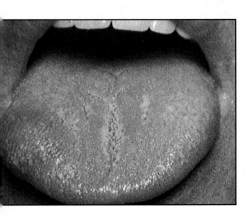

363 Haemangiomas of the tongue. These may be chance findings and are usually innocuous. If large and giving rise to bleeding, laser surgery is the most effective present treatment.

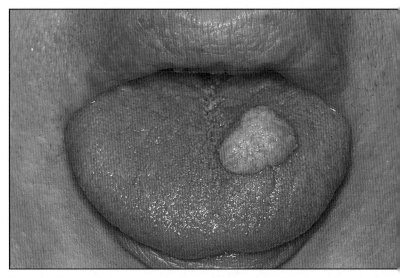

364 Papilloma of the tongue. Benign lesions of the tongue are common, and are either sessile or pedunculated, as in this case. Simple excision under local anaesthetic with biopsy is required.

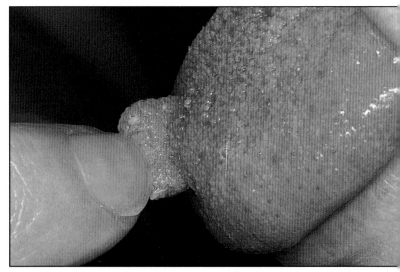

365 Papilloma of the tongue.

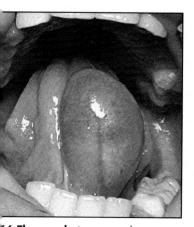

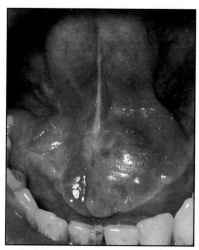

367 Ranula. A ranula, less well-defined, occupying the floor of the mouth.

66 The ranula is a mucocele occur-
ng in the floor of the mouth. A blue
lour and the profunda vein stretched
ross the surface are characteristic. This
nula may extend into the tissues of the
or of the mouth and neck (plunging
nula). Total surgical removal is difficult
cause of the thin wall, and marsup-
isation, as with the lip lesion (see **335**),
adequate treatment. Recurrence is not
common.

The ranula may also present more in the
or of the mouth than on the under-
face of the tongue, and the diagnosis
ty not be so obvious.

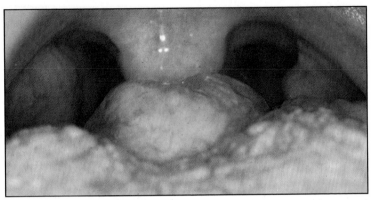

368 Lingual thyroid. Developmental anomalies in the thyroid gland may result in thyroid tissue remaining at the foramen caecum or in the thyroglossal tract. The symptom-free swelling at the base of this tongue is thyroid tissue, and was shown on a radio-active iodine scan to be active. No thyroid gland was palpable in the neck, and there was no iodine uptake other than at the base of the tongue. This lingual thyroid, therefore, was this patient's only active thyroid tissue.

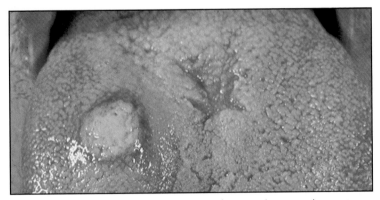

369 Tongue ulceration. The site and type of tongue ulcers give the provisional diagnosis: a margin ulcer with a raised edge is probably a carcinoma; an ulcer on the dorsum with a punched-out margin may be a gumma. Tuberculosis may be the cause of a tender ulcer of the tip of the tongue in an area where tuberculosis is prevalent. However, these clinical findings are only guides. Biopsy of this ulcer on the dorsum showed it to be a solitary aphthous ulcer.

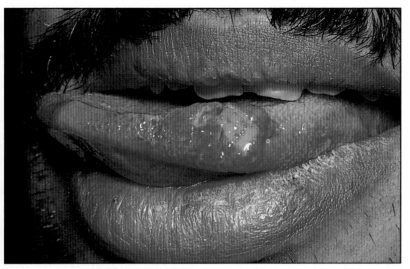

370 An aphthous tongue ulcer of the tongue may be deceptive. A buccal mucosal aphthous ulcer is flat, but on the tongue some swelling due to trauma may make a biopsy necessary in order to be certain of the diagnosis.

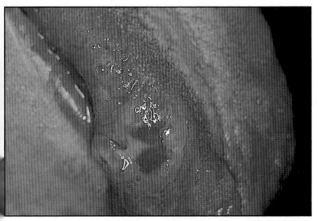

371 Chancre. Tongue ulceration from primary syphilis—a chancre.

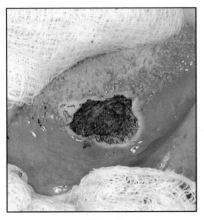

372 Laser excision of a tongue lesion. This shows the minimal reaction at the excision margin, and the non-bleeding base of the excision.

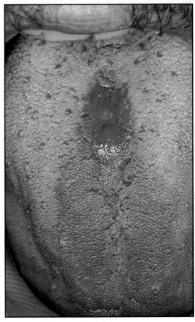

373 Median rhomboid glossitis. This rare anomaly results from failure of the lateral halves of the tongue to fuse posteriorly, leaving the tuberculum impar in the mid-line. A smooth, red, usually symptom-free area persists.

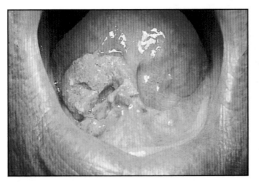

374 Carcinoma of the tongue. This usually occurs on the margin or from the extension of an ulcer on the floor of the mouth (as shown here). Biopsy of this prolifer-ative ulcer showed squamous-cell carcinoma. Partial glossectomy in continuity with a neck dissection, or radio-therapy, are the current treatments.

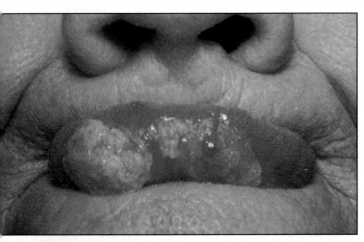

375 Leucoplakia. This is precarcinomatous on the tongue. It may be second-ary to dental or dietary irritation. Leucoplakia is also characteristic of tertiary syphilis, and the tongue is a site where the spirochaete predisposes to carcinoma. Leucoplakia, particularly with no apparent underlying traumatic cause, should be biopsied to exclude carcinoma.

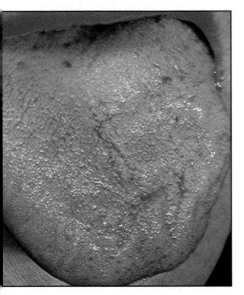

376 Hypoglossal nerve paralysis. Initially, there is fibril-lation, and later, atrophy of the muscles on one side of the tongue. The tongue deviates on protrusion to the side of the nerve palsy. A destructive lesion in the jugular foramen region may extend to involve the hypoglossal nerve as it emerges from the nearby an-terior condylar foramen. This par-alysis of the tongue shows wrinkling caused by fibrillation, and is due to a glomus jugulare tumour, which has also damaged the cranial nerves emerging through the jug-ular foramen (IXth, Xth and XIth).

The hypoglossal nerve, if involved in cervical metastases, may be sectioned in a radial neck dissection.

THE FAUCES AND THE TONSILS

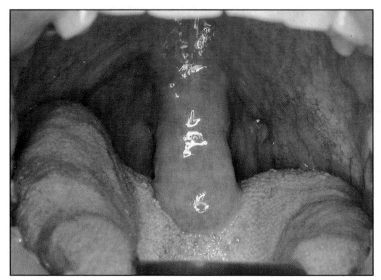

377 The uvula. This obvious anatomical feature in the oropharynx has little pathological significance. When particularly long, however, as here, it has on occasion been thought responsible for various throat symptoms such as discomfort and snoring. Partial amputation has been recommended.

The uvula is excised along with part of the tonsillar fauces and soft palate in the operation of **uvulopalatoplasty** for snoring. The appearance of the palate after operation is seen in **418**.

Snoring

Persistent loud snoring may not only be a social problem, but may predispose to cardiovascular and respiratory problems. Sleep studies are necessary to exclude prolonged episodes of absent breathing (**sleep apnoea**). During sleep studies, monitors make a number of recordings including O_2 and CO_2 levels, pulse rate, respiration rate, ECG, etc. In many instances of sleep apnoea, if the snoring is related to palatal abnormalities such as an elongated uvula and large tonsils, symptoms are relieved by uvulopalatoplasty, which includes tonsillectomy.

Snoring is probably rarely related solely to elongation of the uvula, but is extremely common. In most cases it is tiresome but trivial, and is accentuated by lesions causing obstruction in the upper respiratory tract. Snoring is conspicuous in children with obstruction from the bulk of tonsillar and adenoid lymphoid tissue. The noise from snoring is produced by laxity and vibration of the oropharyngeal muscles. Obesity and excess alcohol are two relevant factors, and frequently attention to these will reduce snoring. Gross snoring, however, may be associated with the ***sleep apnoea syndrome***, and when periods of apnoea occur at night with daytime somnolence, ***sleep studies*** are indicated. These may show significant variations in blood oxygen and CO_2 levels along with variations in cardiac and respiratory rates.

Cor pulmonale may occur in children with grossly obstructing tonsil and adenoid lymphoid tissue. Prolific adult snoring may require an uvulopalatoplasty operation, in which the muscle and overlying mucosa of the palate and fauces are reduced, shortening the palate. The uvula is excised and the tonsils, if present, are removed.

This treatment for snoring is indicated mainly when the snorer is at risk, rather than for the benefit of the one who listens and laser surgery is being appraised for this procedure.

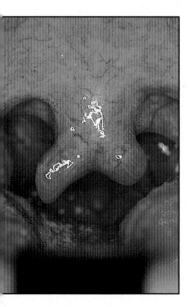

378 Bifid uvula. A common minor congenital deformity of the palate.

It is of little significance, but it may be associated with a submucous palatal cleft. Inflamma-tion of the uvula as an isolated entity may occur, however, and a cherry-like enlarge-ment may be the sole presenting sign of a sore throat.

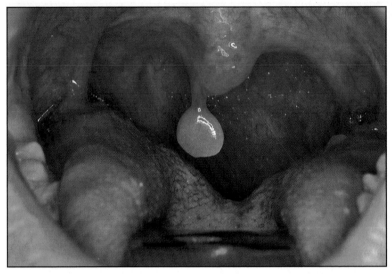

379 Papillomas. These may occur on the uvula, fauces and tonsil. The patient often notices these papillomas when looking at the throat, or they are found at medical examination. Symptoms are uncommon. They are usually pedunculated and are easily and painlessly removable in outpatients. They should be sent for histology to exclude a squamous carcinoma. If ignored, a papilloma may cause symptoms on account of size (**380**).

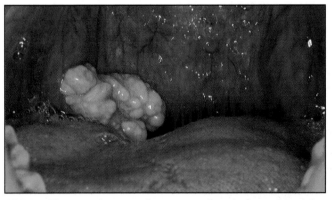

380 Papilloma. A large papilloma arising from the base of the right tonsil.

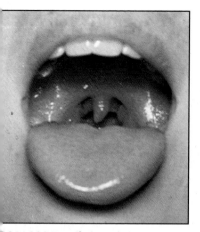
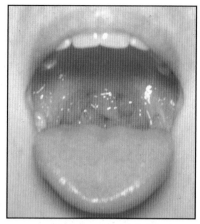

381, 382 Tonsil size. There is no recognised 'normal' size for a tonsil. It is, therefore, arguable as to whether tonsils can be described as 'enlarged'. The apparent size of the tonsil can be altered considerably when the tongue is protruded forcibly. This child, whose oropharynx looks normal when the tongue is slightly protruded, can make the tonsils meet in the mid-line with maximum protrusion of the tongue.

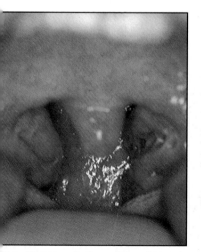
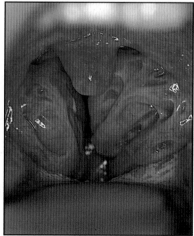

383, 384 Tonsil size affected by tongue depressor. The tongue depressor also alters the apparent size of the tonsils. If the tongue is firmly depressed, the patient gags and the tonsils meet in the mid-line.

177

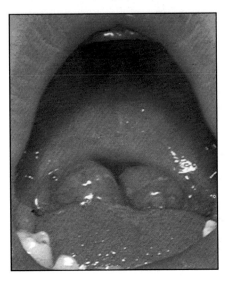

385 Tonsils meeting in the mid-line. It is unusual for tonsils to meet in the mid-line or to overlap, as in this case. Lymphoid tissue of this bulk, particularly during an acute tonsillitis, may cause respir-atory obstruction and severe dysphagia. There is an increased awareness of the severity of upper respiratory tract obstruction from the bulk of tonsillar and adenoic lymphoid tissue. In children, particu-larly at times of superimposed tonsil-litis, the interference with breathing becomes alarming, and obstructive sleep apnoea syndrome is now well-recognised as an important indication for surgery to remove the tonsils and adenoids. Cor pulmonale is seen in children with marked upper respir-atory tract obstruction.

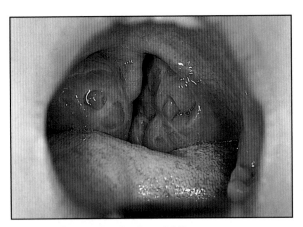

386 Tonsils meeting in the mid-line.

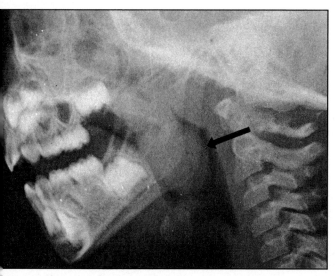

187 Lateral x-ray of tonsils. The tonsils and adenoids show on lateral x-ray (*arrow*), and the soft tissue shadow helps in assessing the degree of obstruc-ion that the lymphoid tissue may be causing. The lingual tonsil is usually large in Down's syndrome patients and contributes to their characteristic bulky tongue.

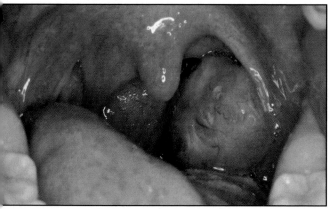

188 Unilateral tonsil enlargement. A tonsil can be described as 'large' when compared with the other tonsil. A conspicuously large tonsil in the absence of acute inflammation is an important finding suggesting either chronic quinsy or a lymphosarcoma. A persistent and conspicuously large tonsil, therefore, should be removed for histology.

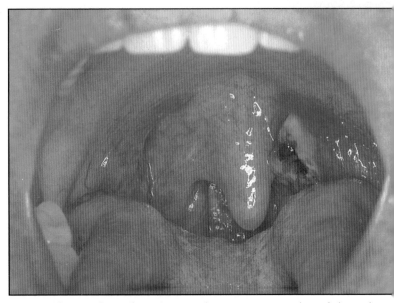

389 A palate and tonsil carcinoma. This presents as an indurated ulcer rather than a diffuse enlargement, and causes referred ear pain. The biopsy is taken from the ulcer margin.

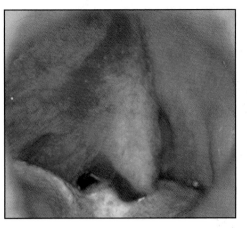

390 Simulated tonsil enlargement. A tonsil may appear to be enlarged by medial displacement from a parapharyngeal swelling, and careful examination of the fauces ensures the the correct diag-nosis is made. is possible to biopsy a normal tonsil and realise later that medial displacement is simulating enlargement. In this case, the parapharyn-geal mass is an internal carotid aneurysm. The initial diagnosis in Casualty would a quinsy—a dangerous error followed by incision.

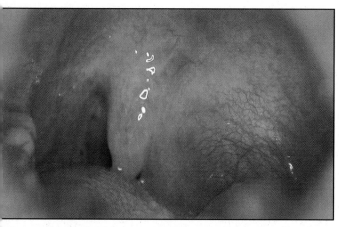

391 Tumours of the deep lobe of the parotid gland causing medical displacement of the tonsil are other more common parapharyngeal swelling, as are chemodectomas, neurofibromata and enlargement of the parapharyngeal lymph nodes.

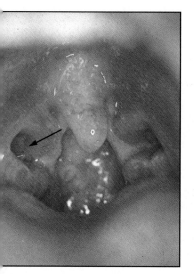

392 Supratonsillar cleft. This recess near the superior pole of the tonsil, if large, tends to collect debris. A mass of yellow fetid material can be extruded from the tonsil with pressure; discomfort or halitosis are symptoms with which this condition may present. Tonsillectomy may be necessary. The surgeon, however, must beware of tonsillectomy for halitosis.

Although dental or gastric pathology may cause this symptom (as may a pharyngeal pouch), the symptom may be imagined by the patient, or by another person complaining about the halitosis.

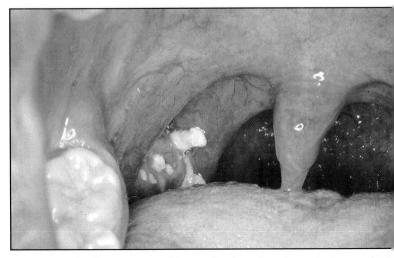

393 Keratosis pharyngeus. Yellow spicules due to hyperkeratinized areas of epithelium are sometimes extensive over the tonsil and lingual tonsil. It is usually a chance finding, and it is important in diagnosis to probe the tonsil (see **394**) to be certain that these yellow areas are not exudate. No treatment is required for this condition unless it is associated with tonsillitis.

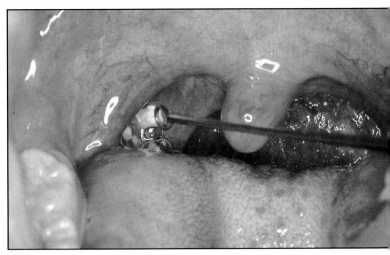

394 Keratosis pharyngeus.

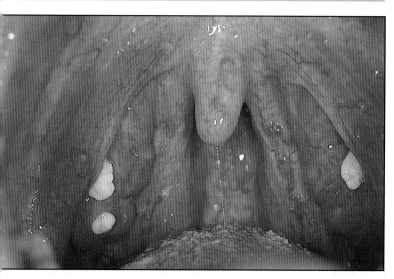

5 Tonsillar exudate. Exudate from tonsillar crypts may appear indistinguishable ⌐n keratosis pharyngeus, and hence palpation with a probe is necessary.

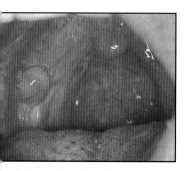 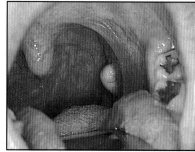

6, 397 Retention cysts. These are common on the tonsil and appear as sessile ⌐ow swellings. If small they can be ignored, and although symptoms are uncommon, a ⌐cern by the patient or a sensation of a lump in the throat may call for surgical ⌐oval. Retention cysts are also seen following tonsillectomy in the region of the fauces ⌐**7**, right).

INFECTIONS OF THE TONSILS, PHARYNX AND OROPHARYNX

Acute tonsillitis

This condition is characterised by sore throat, dysphagia and pyrexia. T appearance of the tonsils varies. An obviously purulent exudate covering t tonsils is common, and is either diffuse or punctate (**398, 399**). An apparen less severely infected throat with hyperaemia of the tonsils only may, howev be associated with severe symptoms. The tonsillar lymph nodes near the an; of the mandible are large and tender.

With acute tonsillitis, the exudate and hyperaemia are centred on the tonsi In an acute pharyngitis, as may be associated with a head cold, the muco membrane of the entire oropharynx is hyperaemic. The gonoccoccus may cau acute pharyngitis, and a throat swab must be placed in Stewart's medium laboratory examination if this infection is suspected. The throat swab in acu tonsillitis commonly grows the haemolytic streptococcus, and a course of o penicillin (often supplemented with an initial intramuscular injection) is invaria curative. An analgesic may also be needed, but lozenges and gargles are usua unnecessary.

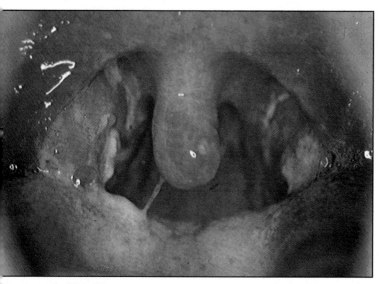

8 Acute tonsillitis. The appearance of the tonsils in acute tonsillitis is either
ᴜse (as above) or punctate (**399**).

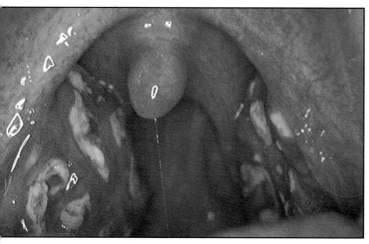

9 Acute tonsillitis (punctate).

Quinsy

This is a complication of acute tonsillitis in which a peritonsillar abscess for
The symptoms may be extremely severe, with absolute dysphagia and p
referred to the ear and trismus, as well as malaise, fever and marked swellin
the tonsillar lymph node. Examination shows the signs of acute tonsillitis w
medial displacement of the tonsils to the mid-line.

If the abscess is pointing, incision at the site marked releases the pus. Since
advent of antibiotics, there is less need for incision of quinsies. High dose
intramuscular penicillin for five days followed by a further five-day course of c
penicillin is the treatment. A large tonsil with medial displacement will per
with inadequate treatment, representing a chronic quinsy in which recurrenc
an acute episode is common. A throat swab of the pus is taken at the tim
diagnosis, and the result may later require changing the penicillin to anot
antibiotic.

A quinsy is extremely rare in children and is also rarely bilateral. Complicati
are uncommon, but bleeding from a quinsy is an important and serious sign;
due to erosion by the peritonsillar pus of one of the adjacent vessels—either
of the tonsillar arteries or the internal carotid artery (***bleeding quinsy***). Quin
not infrequently occur in those who have suffered previous episodes of ac
tonsillitis. Tonsillectomy, which is indicated after a quinsy, is delayed four to
weeks until the acute phase has passed. Vascular fibrous tissue found latera
the tonsil after a quinsy make tonsillectomy technically difficult, and so
advocate tonsillectomy at the time of the acute quinsy (***quinsy tonsillectom***

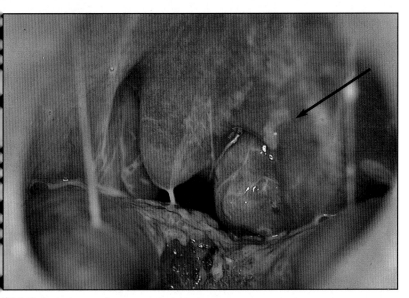

400 Quinsy (arrowed)**.**

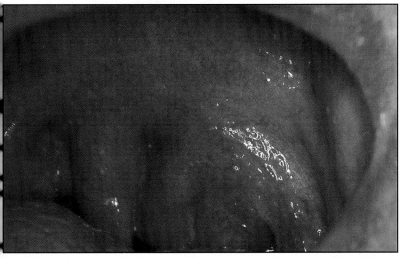

401 Quinsy.

Infectious mononucleosis

Infectious mononucleosis should be suspected if a sore throat and malaise persist despite antibiotic treatment, and a white cell analysis and Paul –Bunnell test are indicated.

A white membrane covering one or both tonsils is characteristic and helpful in diagnosis. Hypersensitivity to ampicillin is increased in infectious mononucleosis, and the antibiotic should be avoided as a severe urticaria follows its use. The positive Paul–Bunnell blood test is diagnostic of infectious mononucleosis, and atypical mononuclear white cells are increased on the blood film.

402

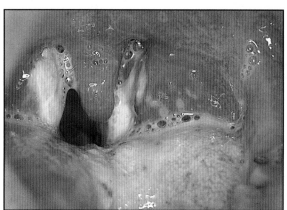

403

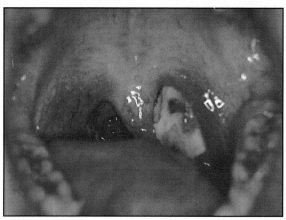

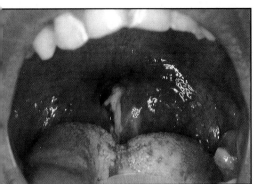

402–404 Infectious mononucleosis.

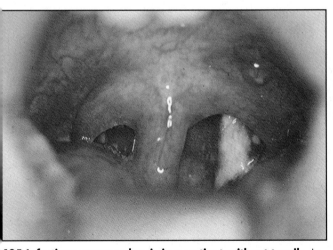

405 Infectious mononucleosis in a patient without tonsils. In this case, the membrane characteristic of infectious mononucleosis is seen either on the lingual tonsil or, as in this case, on a prominent posterior pharyngeal band of lymphoid tissue. A similar white membrane also covers the lymphoid tissue in the post-nasal space; the appearance on examination of the post-nasal space may lead to a suspicion of neoplasm. The increase in bulk of the adenoids also caused a 'nasal voice', which is sometimes characteristic of infectious mononucleosis.

Oral candidiasis (thrush)

Monilia or oral candidiasis (thrush) is one of the fungal infections of the pharynx. Extensive white areas cover the entire oropharynx, and are not confined to the tonsil. They are either continuous (**406**) or punctate (**407**). A swab shows *Candida albicans* and confirms the diagnosis. The condition responds to antifungal mouth washes or lozenges containing nystatin or amphotericin. It is commoner in neonates, and may complicate treatment with broad spectrum antibiotics. Oral candidiasis is one of the commonest upper respiratory tract manifestations of AIDS; unexplained oral fungal infection should make the possibility of AIDS a diagnostic consideration (**408**). Nasal vestibulitis and cervical lymphadenopathy may be associated findings.

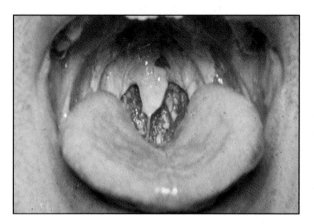

406 Oral candidiasis. Extensive continuous white areas covering the oropharynx.

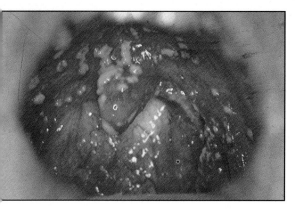

407 Oral candidiasis. Extensive punctate white areas covering the oropharynx.

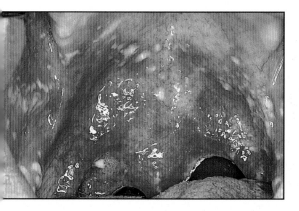

408 AIDS-linked oral candidiasis.

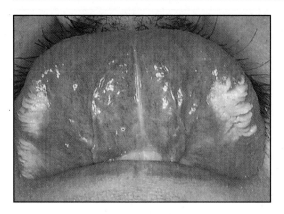

409 Hairy leuco-plakia. Oral candidiasis is the commonest presentation in the pharynx of AIDS, but hairy leucoplakia is a further presentation, along with cervical lymphadenopathy.

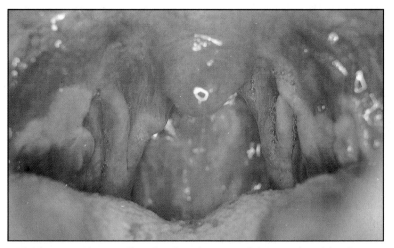

410 Ulcers on the tonsil and soft palate. *Candida* was cultured, but these are *snail-track ulcers of secondary syphilis*.

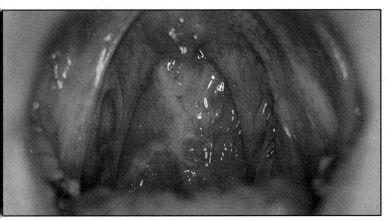

411 Chronic pharyngitis. In this condition there is a generalised hyperaemia of the pharyngeal mucous membrane, with hyperaemic masses of lymphoid tissue on the posterior wall of the oropharynx. A persistent, slightly sore throat is the main symptom. The cause is usually 'irritative' rather than due to chronic infection. Environment, occupation, diet and tobacco are the common factors.

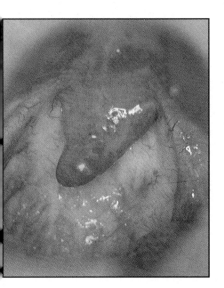

412 Scleroma with scarring of the soft palate and oropharynx. This is a specific chronic inflammatory disease of the upper respiratory tract mucosa predominantly occurring in Eastern Europe, Asia and South America. A protracted painless inflammation of the nose (***rhinoscleroma***), pharynx or larynx is followed after many years by extensive scarring, which is particularly apparent in the oropharynx. Unlike gummatous ulceration, which is a differential diagnosis, scleroma is not destructive; the uvula is preserved, although it may be retracted by scarring into the nasopharynx, and is seen with the post-nasal mirror. The histology of the mucosa in scleroma is characteristic and diagnostic.

TONSILLECTOMY

Tonsillectomy is one of the most frequently performed operations in the world. Stricter indications for operating, however, are reducing the number of tonsillectomies. Recurrent episodes of acute tonsillitis, interfering with school or work, are the main indications. A quinsy or chronic tonsillitis are other indications, along with marked enlargement interfering with the airway.

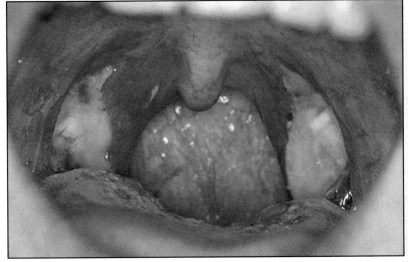

413 The tonsillar fossae following tonsillectomy. These are covered with a white/yellow membrane for about 10 days until the fossae are epithelialised.

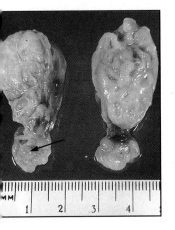

414 Tonsils after removal to demonstrate the lingual pole (*arrow*). The pole must be included at tonsillectomy. A tonsil remnant may be left inadvertently at this site, giving rise to further infection, but tonsils do not 're-grow'.

Adenoid tissue is, however, not possible to enucleate and remove *in toto*; it may recur, particularly when removed before four years of age.

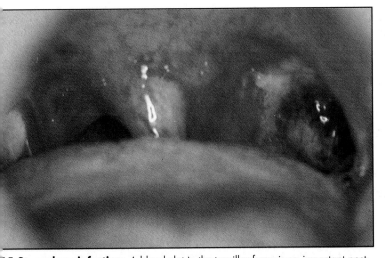

415 Secondary infection. A blood clot in the tonsillar fossa is an important postoperative finding, and almost certainly indicates secondary infection. This occurs between the third and 10th day, and is associated with bleeding and increased pain. The bleeding is usually scanty and settles when antibiotics control the secondary infection. Severe delayed bleeding after tonsillectomy may occur, however; the finding of a blood clot in a tonsillar fossa must not be ignored.

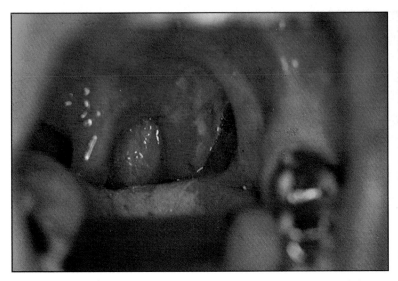

416 Secondary tonsillar infection with bleeding and bruising of the soft palate. This appearance may be related to an excessively traumatic tonsillectomy. An infected blood clot is present in the tonsillar fossa; removal may cause more bleeding. A tonsillar blood clot present with primary bleeding, however, should be removed if possible; this may settle the bleeding.

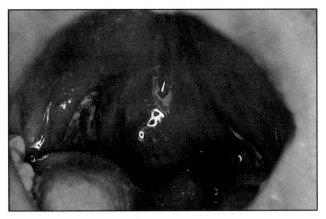

417 Secondary tonsillar infection with bleeding and bruising of the soft palate.

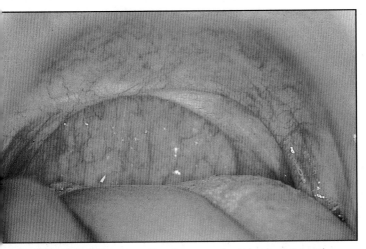

18 Guillotine tonsillectomy. Tonsillectomy today is by dissection with inimal injury to the fauces and surrounding structures. Adept use of the guillotine ay also be a rapid and effective surgical technique, but removal of the uvula nd fauces is possible in inexperienced hands. Fortunately, post-operative scaring of the palate and uvula is frequently symptom-free. This appearance of the oft palate with conspicuous shortening is similar to that following the **uvulo-alatoplasty** operation for severe snoring.

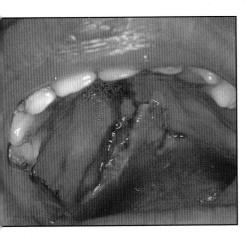

419 Palatal trauma. Lacerations to the hard and soft palate are not uncommon. The oft-given advice to children not to 'run with a pencil or similar object in their mouth' is intended to off-set palatal laceration resulting from a fall. Suturing, however, is usually unnecessary, and unless there is gross mucosal separation, the palate and tongue heal well spontaneously following trauma.

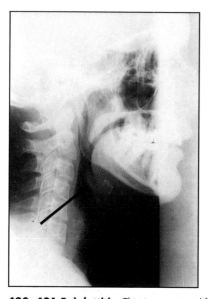 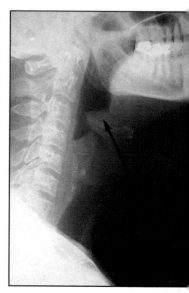

420, 421 Epiglottitis. This is a serious, life-threatening condition and a diagnosis that may be missed. The complaint of a sore throat in an ill patient with a history of dysphagia and fever, often strongly suggestive of a quinsy, *is associated with little amiss on oral examination*. Such a situation strongly suggests epiglottitis, and a lateral soft-tissue x-ray is frequently diagnostic.

The normal narrow contour of the epiglottis is seen to be replaced by a round swelling (*arrows*). This condition, if ignored, may lead to stridor, respiratory obstruction and death if the airway is occluded.

Early diagnosis, hospital admission and intravenous antibiotic (e.g. cefuroxime) therapy is curative. Close nursing observation of the airway is necessary.

THE LARYNX

INFLAMMATION OF THE LARYNX

Laryngitis

Whether acute or chronic, laryngitis presents with hoarseness and generalised hyperaemia of the laryngeal mucous membrane. *Acute laryngitis* commonly follows an upper respiratory tract infection, or is traumatic following vocal abuse (see **434**). Voice rest is the most effective treatment.

   Chronic laryngitis may be associated with infection in the upper or lower respiratory tract, but is commonly 'irritative' due to occupation and environment, vocal abuse or tobacco. The unusual laryngitis of *myxoedema* must not be forgotten.

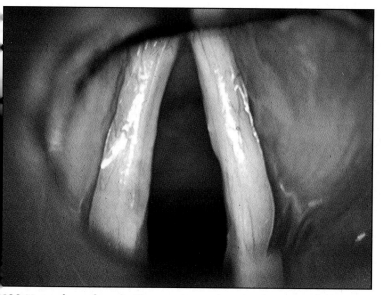

422 Normal vocal cords. These are ivory coloured and smooth with few vessels on the surface. This is the view obtained through a laryngoscope at direct microlaryngoscopy.

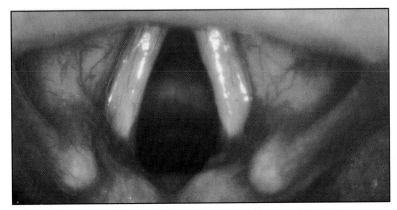

423 A fibreoptic endoscopic view of a normal larynx (see **67**).

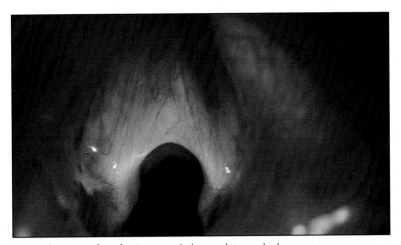

424 A laryngeal web. Congenital abnormalities or the larynx are uncommon. Webbing of varying degrees of severity is one of the commoner developmental abnormalities, and presents as hoarseness. Similar webbing may follow inadvertent trauma at endoscopic surgery to both vocal cords near the anterior commissure. A mucosal web is treated with surgical division. Most webs, however, are deep and fibrous and need an indwelling 'keel' after division to avoid recurrence.

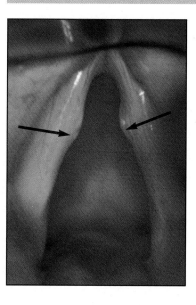

425 Laryngeal nodules (*arrows*). A specific and localised type of chronic laryngitis, often seen in professional voice users, is laryngeal nodules (***singers' nodules***).

Initially an oedema is seen on the vocal cord between the anterior one-third and posterior two-thirds of the cord. Removal of the nodules may be necessary, but attention to the underlying voice production by a speech therapist is the most important aspect of treatment.

These nodules are not an uncommon cause of hoarseness in children, particularly of large families involved in competitive shouting (***screamers' nodules***). Vocal cord nodules are also seen in those who overuse or misuse their voices.

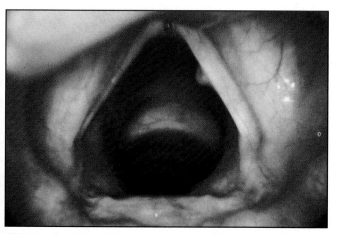

426 Vocal cord nodule seen through a fibreoptic endoscope.
A solitary vocal cord nodule at the characteristic site is not uncommon, although they are usually bilateral and fairly symmetrical.

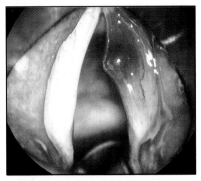

427 Vocal cord nodule with haematoma. A vocal cord nodule with haematoma formation following vocal abuse.

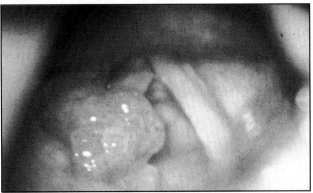

428 Juvenile papilloma.

Juvenile papillomas are most important to exclude in a hoarse child or baby, for if the hoarseness is ignored, stridor will develop, since the papillomas extend to occlude the lumen of the larynx. ('Screamers' nodules [laryngeal nodules], however, are the commonest cause of hoarseness in children.)

In this curious condition, multiple wart-like excrescences develop, usually before the age of five, on or around the vocal cords. Recurrence follows removal, but fortunately eventual spontaneous regression is usual. The cause is now established as the human papillomavirus.

Management consists of regular microlaryngoscopy with removal of the papillomas using the carbon dioxide laser. A tracheostomy may be necessary, but should be avoided if possible, as papillomas tend to develop around the tracheal opening and 'seed' further down the tracheo-bronchial tree. In severe cases, chemotherapy with interferon is currently being evaluated.

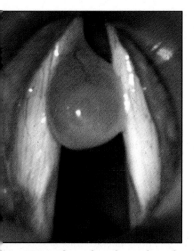 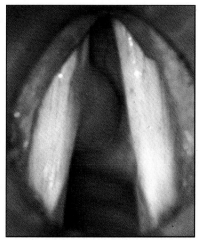

29, 430 Pedunculated vocal cord polyp. A large pedunculated polyp may form ↧ the vocal cord and be missed on examination for it moves above and below the cord ↧ expiration and inspiration. A large polyp (**429**, left) is less apparent (**430**, right) ↧hen it is below the cord on inspiration.

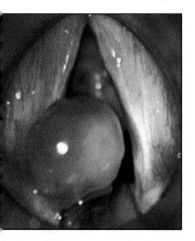

431 Intubation granulomas of the larynx. These result from trauma by the anaesthetic tube to the mucosa overlying the vocal process of the arytenoid; they are, therefore, posterior. With the skill that anaesthetists have achieved for endo-tracheal intubation, trauma to this region is uncommon.

Granulomas at this site also develop after prolonged vocal abuse has caused a chronic laryngitis in which the epithelium over the vocal process becomes ulcerated ('contact ulcers'). Removal at the pedicle is necessary.

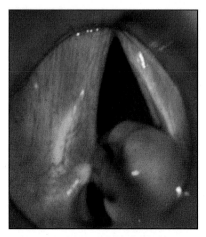

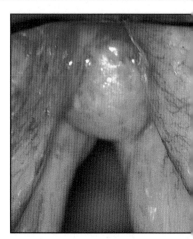

432 Granuloma of the larynx excision. Here the pedicle of the intubation granuloma is being held with forceps prior to removal. Recurrence frequently follows excision, but laser beam techniques appear to lessen the likelihood. Relatively large lesions can occupy the posterior half of the larynx with minimal voice change. Anteriorly in the larynx, however, small lesions cause conspicuous voice change.

433 Polyp at the anterior commissure. This site is not always easy to see on indirect laryngoscopy for it may be partly obscured by the tubercle of the epiglottis. The laryngoscope is placed against the tubercle, displacing it forwards and a clear view is obtained.

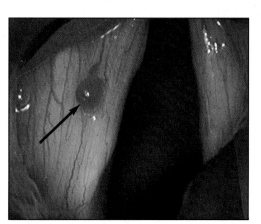

434 Haemangiomas. These are uncommon vocal cord lesions and if small may cause no hoarseness or bleeding, and be a chance finding on examination. Laser surgery promises to be the effective treatment for larger haemangiomas.

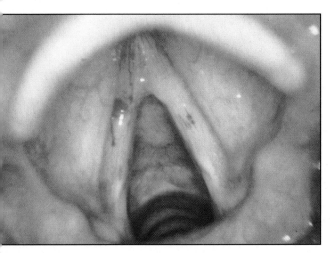

435 Acute laryngitis showing slight hyperaemia and oedema of both vocal cords seen with the fibreoptic endoscope.

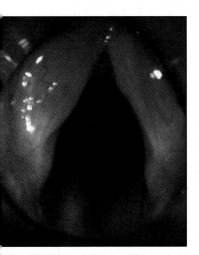 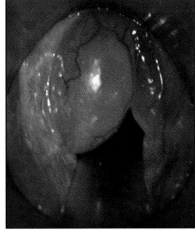

436, 437 Chronic laryngitis. With this condition, hyperaemia of the mucous membrane may be associated with other changes in the larynx. Oedema of the margin of the vocal cords is common (Reinke's oedema), so that the free margin is polypoid and a large sessile polyp may form. The oedema, although affecting both cords, may be more marked on one side.

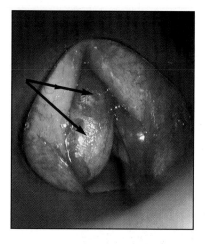

438 Hypertrophy of the ventricular bands. Hypertrophy of the ventricular bands is another finding in chronic laryngitis and they may meet in the mid-line on phonation, producing a characteristic hoarseness. Reinke's oedema is also present. Microlaryngoscopy and surgical excision of the oedematous margins is effective with dissection or the laser beam. Excision to the anterior commissure is made on one cord only to avoid webbing.

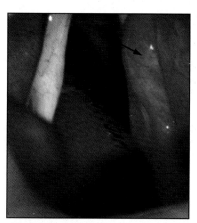

439 Prolapse of the ventricular mucous membrane. This may also occur in chronic laryngitis and presents as a supraglottic swelling. A supraglottic cyst or carcinoma must be excluded.

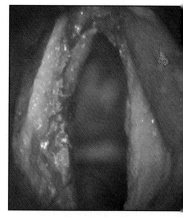

440 Long-standing chronic laryngitis. The mucous membrane may become extremely hypertrophic with white patches (leucoplakia). Histologically, the white patches represent areas of keratosis which may precede malignant change and be reported as carcinoma *in situ*. This patient had smoked over 60 cigarettes a day for 50 years.

NEOPLASMS OF THE LARYNX

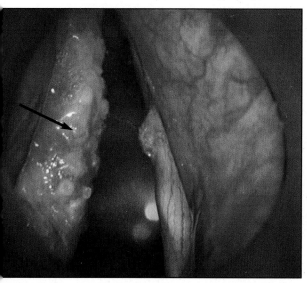

41 Carcinoma of the vocal cord. This usually occurs in smokers. The indurated leucoplakia on this vocal cord *(arrow)* is a well-differentiated squamous-cell carcinoma that has arisen as a result of chronic laryngitis with hyperkeratosis.

The prognosis for vocal cord carcinoma with radiotherapy is excellent, with a cure rate of over 90% for early lesions. The voice returns to normal, as does the appearance of the vocal cord.

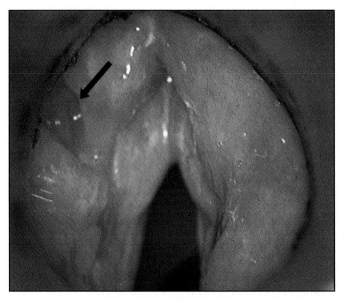

442 Supraglottic squamous-cell carcinoma. Carcinoma of the larynx commonly involves the vocal cord (glottic carcinoma), but lesions may develop below the cord (subglottic) or above the cord (supraglottic). The ulcerated area of granulation tissue above the oedematous vocal cord in this case is a squamous-cell carcinoma.

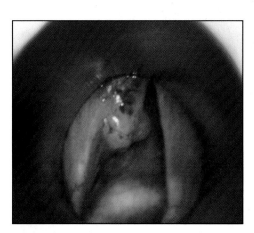

443 Subglottic squamous-cell carcinoma. The prognosis for supraglottic and subglottic carcinoma is worse than for glottic carcinoma; for hoarseness is delayed until the cord is involved and the greater vascularity and lymphatic drainage above and below the cord predisposes to earlier metastasis.

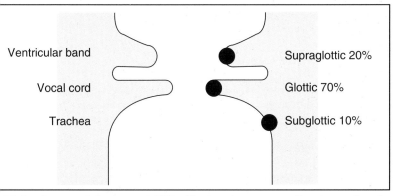

Ventricular band — Supraglottic 20%

Vocal cord — Glottic 70%

Trachea — Subglottic 10%

44 Carcinoma of the larynx. 70% of laryngeal carcinomas affect the vocal cord.

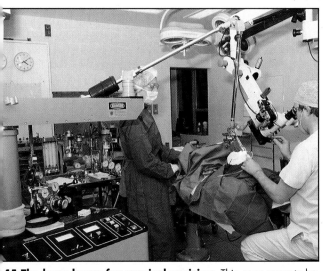

45 The laser beam for surgical excision. This may prove to be the technique of choice for certain lesions in the upper respiratory tract. In this case it is being used at microlaryngoscopy to excise an intubation granuloma (see **431**). The laser is now widely used for the removal of tongue (see **372**) and pharyngeal lesions, particularly haemangiomas and other vascular lesions. The laser also appears to have advantages for excision of juvenile papillomas, intubation granulomas and possibly laryngeal webs. Use of the operating microscope ensures precise excision with the laser beam, which causes considerably less tissue damage than cautery or diathermy.

LARYNGEAL SURGERY

Laryngectomy

Nearly all cases of early carcinoma of the vocal cord are cured with radiotherapy or laser surgery. Disease, however, may remain with extensive cord carcinoma, with supra- or subglottic lesions, or with carcinoma of the pyriform fossa or epiglottis.

Partial laryngectomy (laryngofissure, extended laryngofissure or supraglottic laryngectomy) gives adequate resection of some laryngeal carcinomas, but frequently a ***total laryngectomy*** is required. This radical surgery, which may be associated with a neck dissection if the nodes are involved, means a permanent tracheostome, and an alternative method of speech has to be developed. Air is swallowed into the upper oesophagus, and coherent speech is achieved by learning to phonate with controlled regurgitation of the air. Even with intensive speech therapy, some patients remain unable to achieve reasonable voice.

Conservative laryngectomy (supraglottic or hemilaryngectomy) aims in the smaller laryngeal cancers to preserve part or all of the vocal cords and to avoid a tracheostome, so that laryngeal voice is preserved. For those who are unable to speak after total laryngectomy, or as a primary procedure with laryngectomy, a valve fitted between the tracheostome and oesophagus enables air to be redirected with a more normal voice production (Blom–Singer valve).

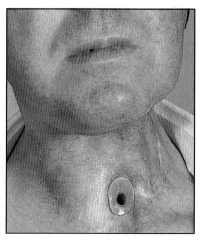

446 Total laryngectomy with left radical neck dissection.

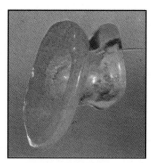

447 Stomal stud. Stenosis of the tracheostome is sometimes a post-operative problem, and a small stomal stud can be used.

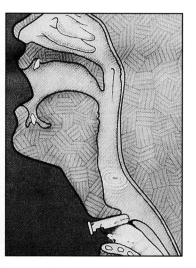

448 The Blom–Singer voice prosthesis shown diagrammatically and positioned into the new opening to the oesophagus at the top of the tracheostome. This prosthesis may be inserted at the time of laryngectomy or placed later in those who are unable to develop coherent speech.

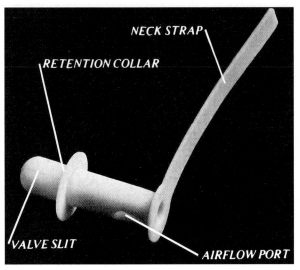

NECK STRAP

RETENTION COLLAR

VALVE SLIT

AIRFLOW PORT

449 Blom–Singer voice prosthesis.

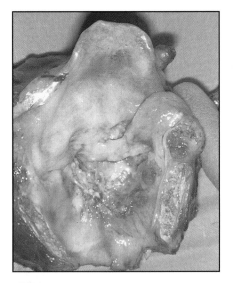

450 Laryngectomy specimen.
This shows a large laryngeal
carcinoma extending above and
below the right vocal cord and across
to the left side of the larynx. It also
shows the hyoid, thyroid and cricoid
cartilages and upper rings of trachea,
which are removed at laryngectomy.

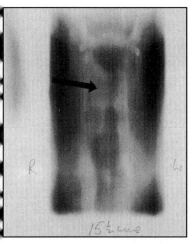

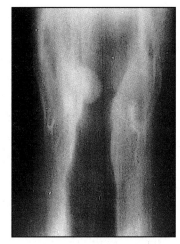

451, 452 Laryngeal tomogram. This x-ray is a helpful investigation to assist definition of tumour extent. **451** (left) shows an extensive carcinoma; **452** (right) shows a large pedunculated supraglottic swelling, which proved to be a fibroma—a rare benign laryngeal tumour.

Hoarseness

Hoarseness may be due to *paralysis of one vocal cord*, the left being more commonly involved. Lack of cord movement on phonation is diagnosed on indirect laryngoscopy or fibreoptic laryngoscopy. Although temporary idiopathic cord palsy is the single most common cause, involvement of the left recurrent laryngeal nerve in chest disease must be excluded. Any hilar lymph node lesion in the region of the aortic arch may involve this nerve, such as secondaries from lung carcinoma. The enlarged left atrium of mitral stenosis may also press on the left recurrent laryngeal nerve and cause hoarseness, as may an aortic aneurysm or the enlarged pulmonary artery of pulmonary hypertension.

The recurrent laryngeal nerves are also occasionally damaged in the neck by severe external injury, or by thyroid carcinoma or surgery. Central lesions, or lesions near the jugular foramen involving the vagus, may also cause cord paralysis, and hoarseness is one of the symptoms of posterior inferior cerebellar artery thrombosis.

Hoarseness, particularly a whispered voice with normal larynx, is a functional voice problem. *Hysterical aphonia* is not uncommon in young women, and stems from a superficial psychiatric upset. Treatment from the *speech therapist* is usually effective without referral to a psychiatrist being necessary. Curious alterations in the voice or hoarseness may also be due to a *hysterical dysphonia*.

Phonosurgery

Microsurgical techniques are effective to restore normal quality of a hoarse voice. Minute lesions on or within the vocal cord can be excised or enucleated with precision.

Phonosurgery is of particular use for established vocal cord palsy. The voice is weak and "breathy" because the glottis does not fully "close" on phonation. Techniques to medialise or increase the bulk of the immobile cord enables full closure of the glottis and a normal or near-normal voice to be achieved.

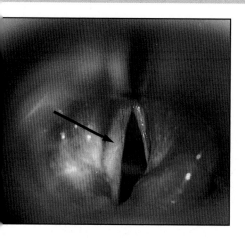

453 Left vocal cord palsy.
The paralysed vocal cord is seen to lie near the mid-line (*arrow*) and undergoes no movement on phonation at indirect laryngoscopy (see **66**).

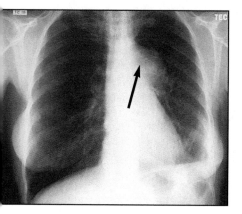

454 X-ray of aortic aneurysm (*arrow*). Pressure on the left recurrent laryngeal nerve causes nerve palsy and hoarseness.

Microsurgery of the larynx

The use of the microscope for direct laryngoscopy has greatly increased the scope and precision of laryngeal surgery. All small benign lesions of the larynx are excised with this technique. Biopsies of malignant disease can be taken accurately from the suspicious area with minimal damage to adjacent tissue.

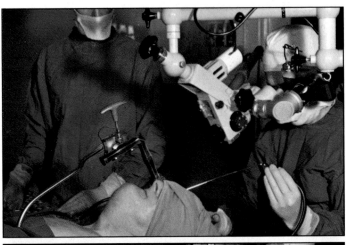

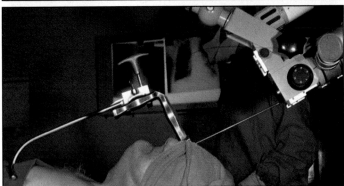

455, 456 Microlaryngoscopy. The holder for the laryngoscope is clamped (**455**, top), enabling the surgeon to have both hands free for instrumentation. The x-rays are seen in the background (**456**, below); the chest x-ray and x-ray of the cervical spine are routine investigations before direct laryngoscopy. Cold light instruments give brighter and more reliable illumination than bulbs, and the development of a light-transmitting glass fibre cable has been another advance in endoscopy.

Tracheostomy

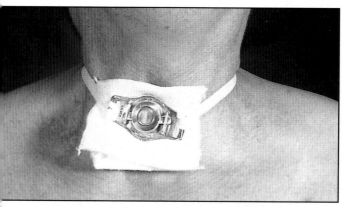

457 A patient after tracheostomy (with speaking valve).

Obstruction of the larynx causes stridor, and may necessitate a tracheostomy. Acute inflammatory conditions of the upper respiratory tract (e.g. epiglottitis), foreign bodies or neoplasms limiting the airway are the commonest causes of stridor.

Tracheostomy is also required for respiratory failure due to central depression of the respiratory centre, e.g. strokes, barbiturate poisoning, head injury, poliomyelitis or tetanus. Multiple rib fractures or severe chest infections may require tracheostomy. Tracheostomy enables breathing to be controlled by an intermittent positive pressure respirator, and bronchial secretions can be removed with suction. A prolonged obstruction of the glottis may occur with juvenile papillomas, severe trauma to the larynx or bilateral cord palsies, making a permanent tracheostomy necessary. *A tracheostomy tube with a speaking valve* allows air to enter during inspiration, but closes on expiration so that air passes through the larynx for phonation.

Emergency tracheostomy may be a difficult operation, particularly if done under local anaesthetic when a general anaesthetic with intubation is not practical. An opening into the trachea through the crico-thyroid membrane offers a simpler and more direct relief for upper respiratory tract obstruction.

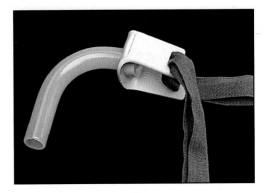

458 Plastic tracheostomy tubes. These are also in common use.

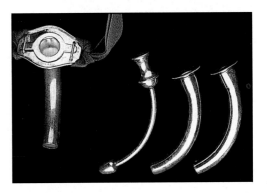

459 Silver trache ostomy tubes in common use (Negus).

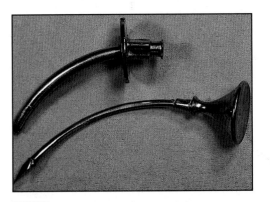

460 Cricothyrotomy cannula with trocar. This instrument has been devised for emergency operations. A tracheostomy can be performed later when the emergency of the acute obstruction is past.

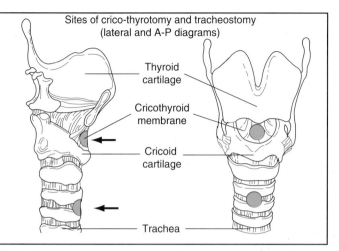

Sites of crico-thyrotomy and tracheostomy
(lateral and A-P diagrams)

Thyroid cartilage

Cricothyroid membrane

Cricoid cartilage

Trachea

461 Tracheostomy. Openings are usually made between the 2nd and 3rd tracheal rings. A 'higher' tracheostomy predisposes to stenosis of the larynx in the subglottic region.

The airway is most accessible and superficial at the level of the cricothyroid membrane, and in acute laryngeal obstruction an opening through this membrane will restore the airway. The cricothyrotomy opening is, however, for emergency, and is only temporary. Indwelling tubes at this site lead to subglottic stenosis of the larynx.

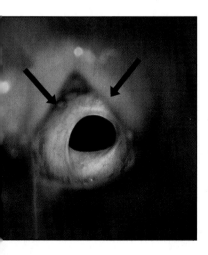

462 Subglottic stenosis. Slightly hyperaemic cords with an area of ring-like stenosis below the vocal cords can be seen in this patient. This stenosis followed trauma, partly related to a road traffic accident in which the trachea was injured, and also related to a high tracheostomy through the first tracheal ring.

Dilation is rarely effective for this type of cicatricial stenosis, and excision of the stenotic area of the trachea with end-to-end anastomosis or grafting procedures are necessary.

Subglottic stenosis is also a complication of prolonged endotracheal intubation.

THE HYPOPHARYNX AND OESOPHAGUS

Globus pharyngeus

This is a very common condition in which the patient, not infrequently a young girl, complains of a sensation of a lump in the throat. The site indicated is the cricoid region.

When taking the history, a helpful direct question is to ask whether the lump is most apparent on swallowing food, fluid or saliva; the patient with globus will consistently reply that saliva is the problem, and that the symptom occurs between meals.

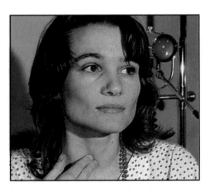

463 Globus pharyngeus. The patient is indicating the region of the cricoid cartilage which is the site of discomfort with globus pharyngeus.

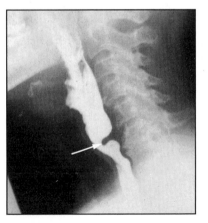

464 Barium swallow. Globus pharyngeus is a psychosomatic condition, but there is a demonstrable spasm of the cricopharyngeus on barium swallow, where the barium column is seen to be 'nipped'. Over-attention by the patient perpetuates the spasm, and usually reassurance and explanation are the only treatments required.

globus pharyngeus does not necessarily occur in hysterics, and 'globus hystericus' is a misnomer. It is also a condition that calls for investigation, particularly in the older age group, when it may be the presenting symptom of disease in the oesophagus or stomach. Hiatus hernia and oesophageal reflux commonly cause cricopharyngeal spasm, and gastric ulcers and neoplasms may also present with globus. A barium swallow and meal is therefore an important investigation (see **464**). Cervical osteoarthritis (**465** and **466**, *arrow*) with marked changes in the region of the 6th cervical vertebra may also give rise to globus.

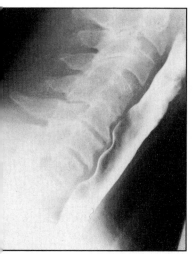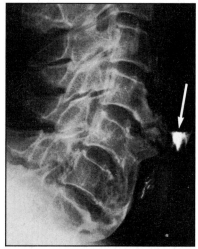

465, 466 Cervical osteoarthritis. Projection of cervical osteophytes into the post-ricoid region of the upper oesophagus causes cricopharyngeal spasm and the symptom of globus. In this x-ray, gross osteophytes have caused 'nipping' of the barium (*arrow*) by the cricopharyngeus muscle.

Pharyngeal pouch

This is a herniation of mucous membrane through the posterior fibres of the inferior constrictor muscle above the cricopharyngeus, usually occurring in old age. The defect predisposing to its development is a failure of coordinated relaxation of the cricopharyngeus on swallowing. A pouch is frequently associated with a hiatus hernia.

A small pouch may cause no symptoms, but when large, dysphagia develops, varying from slight to absolute. There is regurgitation of undigested food, gurgling may be heard in the neck after eating, or a swelling may be seen, laterally in the neck, usually on the left. The pouch accumulates food, and spillage into the respiratory tract may cause coughing. A pouch may present with respiratory disease—either bronchitis, apical fibrosis simulating tuberculosis, or acute pulmonary infection (bronchitis, bronchopneumonia or a lung abscess).

The barium swallow is the only investigation required to confirm the diagnosis of a pharyngeal pouch. If symptoms are marked, excision of the pouch via a neck incision is necessary. Rarely, a carcinoma occurs within the lumen of a pharyngeal pouch.

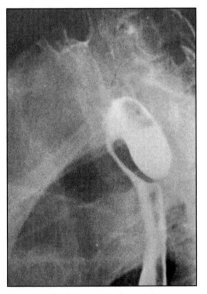 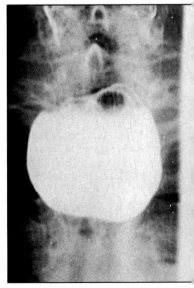

467, 468 Pharyngeal pouch.

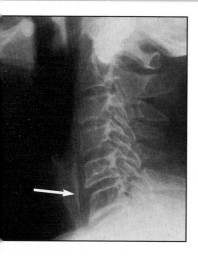

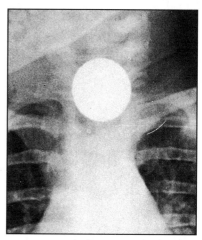

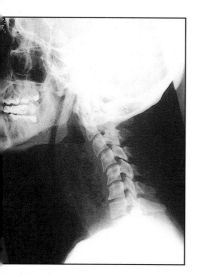

469–471 Foreign bodies in the oesophagus. Foreign bodies, such as bones, coins, pins, dentures and small toys, may impact in the upper third of the oesophagus. A history of possible foreign impaction must not be ignored as oesophageal perforation leads to cervical cellulitis and mediastinitis, which may be fatal.

Air seen on x-ray behind the pharynx and oesophagus is diagnostic of a perforation. Persistent dysphagia, pain referred to the neck or back, pain on inspiration and fever all suggest a foreign body.

Chest x-ray and x-ray of the neck are essential investigations, but even if negative, persistent symptoms are suspicious, and oesophagoscopy is necessary. However, coins which pass the cricopharyngeus usually traverse the rest of the gut, and rarely require removal.

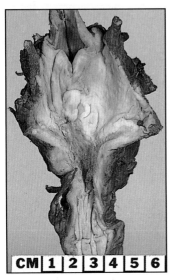 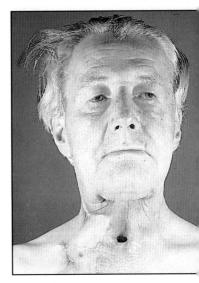

472, 473 Carcinoma of the pyriform fossa and upper oesophagus. The presenting signs are dysphagia for solids and pain, commonly referred to the ear. There is early metastasis to the cervical nodes. A carcinoma involving mainly the medial wall of the pyriform fossa causes hoarseness.

The prognosis is not good, particularly with upper oesophageal carcinoma, whether treatment is with radiotherapy or surgery. Resection for these carcinomas involves a pharyngolaryngectomy and the replacement or reconstruction of the cervical oesophagus poses technical problems. Immediate replacement with stomach or colon, mobilised and brought through the thorax and sutured to the pharynx, is one technique.

The delayed use of neck and chest myocutaneous flaps is an alternative method of reconstruction. Microvascular surgical techniques have enabled immediate reconstruction with a section of the ileum, which is a further option.

Chapter 5

The Head and Neck

SALIVARY GLANDS

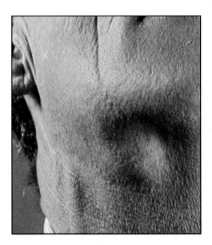

474 Submandibular calculus. A calculus obstructing the submandibular duct causes painful and intermittent enlargement of the gland.

The swelling occurs on eating and regresses slowly. Secondary infection in the gland leads to persistent tender swelling of the gland.

The swelling in the submandibular triangle is visible and palpable bimanually, with one finger in the mouth.

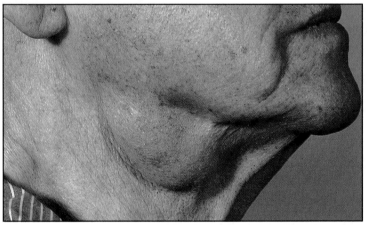

475 Grossly enlarged submandibular gland. This develops if an impacted calculus is ignored.

A neoplasm of the submandibular gland is the differential diagnosis if the enlargement is persistent and there is no evidence of a calculus on x-ray. The nodular surface and the firm, non-tender character on palpation of this gland are also suggestive of a neoplasm, commonly a ***pleomorphic adenoma*** or adenoid cystic carcinoma.

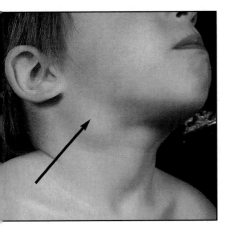

476 Tonsillar lymph node enlargement. A tonsillar lymph node enlargement (*arrow*) may be similar to an enlarged submandibular gland. This node is frequently palpable in children, being more conspicuous at times of ton-sillar or upper respiratory tract infection, and may become very obvious, as in this case. The node is soft and tender.

Exact location of the site is important: it is **posterior to the submandibular triangle** at the angle of the mandible, and not within the submandibular triangle.

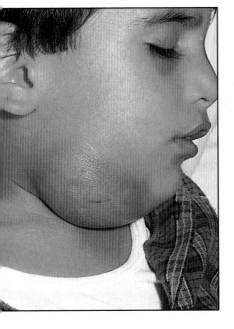

477 Abscess formation in a submandibular triangle lymph node secondary to dental infection. **Mumps** may also cause a tender submandibular swelling, and an enlarged lymph node in the submandibular triangle, secondary to dental infection, simulates gland involvement.

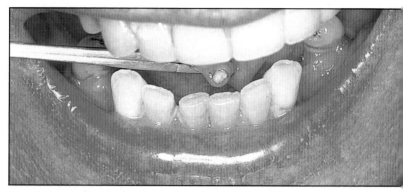

478 Submandibular calculus impacted at the orifice of the duct. This is easily removed with local anaesthesia in the out-patients.

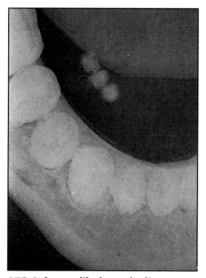

479 Submandibular calculi demonstrated on x-ray impacted in the duct. An anterior calculus may be removed by incision over the duct in the floor of the mouth, a suture being placed posterior to the calculus to prevent "slippage backwards" towards the gland.

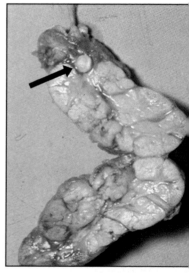

480 Excision of the submandibular gland (specimen) is required for calculi impacted in the duct or within the gland (as demonstrated here).

Care is taken in this operation to preserve the mandibular branch of the facial nerve which crosses the submandibular triangle to supply the muscles of the angle of the mouth.

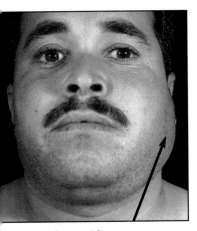

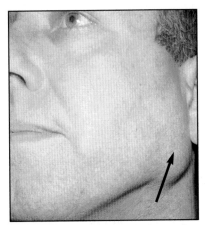

481 Mixed parotid tumour (pleomorphic adenoma) (*arrow*). These present as a firm, smooth, non-tender swelling. The growth is slow, so the history may be long.

The bulk of the parotid lies in the neck posterior to the ramus of the mandible, and parotid tumours do not usually cause predominantly facial swelling.

482 Parotid swelling. A softer swelling in the tail of the parotid (*arrow*) may be an **adenolymphoma** (Warthin's tumour), a benign tumour of salivary gland tissue within a parotid lymph node.

The pleomorphic adenoma is a low-grade malignant tumour, and is commonly in the superficial lobe of the parotid. The treatment is a superficial parotidectomy with preservation of the facial nerve. A soft parotid swelling with a short history and a partial or complete facial palsy is probably an adenoid cystic carcinoma or higher-grade malignant tumour of the parotid gland, requiring total parotidectomy with sacrifice of the facial nerve and radiotherapy.

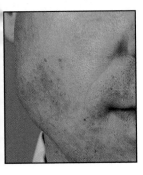

483 Congenital hypertrophy of the masseter muscle. Careful palpation follows observation of a swelling, and what appears as a parotid mass here is palpable as a congenital hypertrophy of the masseter muscle.

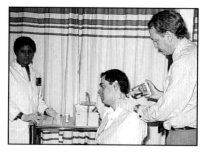

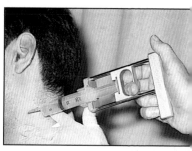

484, 485 A needle aspiration is a frequently used investigation for neck swellings. Aspiration from the neck swelling under local anaesthetic enables histological examination of the aspirate smear to be made. This may avoid the necessity of an incision and "open" biopsy, or biopsy incision of the node.

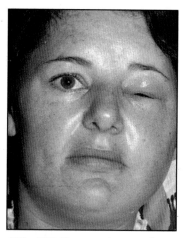

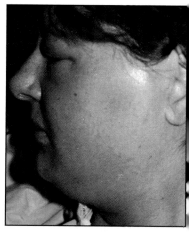

486, 487 Mumps. Acute viral parotitis is a common infection, and the diagnosis is usually obvious.

Well-defined tender swelling of the parotid gland, first on one side and shortly after on the other, with associated trismus and malaise, are characteristic. However, mumps can be deceptive when it remains unilateral and the swelling is not strictly confined to the parotid. In this case of mumps, the swelling involved the side of the face, causing lid and facial oedema. **Unilateral total deafness is a complication of mumps.**

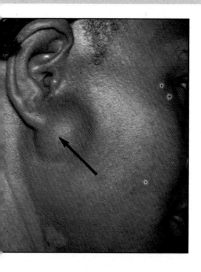

488 Sebaceous cyst. A swelling in the parotid region (*arrow*), but on the face suggests another diagnosis. There is a small punctum on the swelling in this picture, diagnostic of a sebaceous cyst.

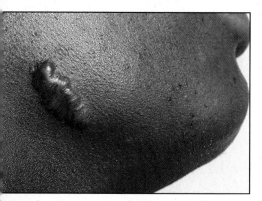

489 Sebaceous cyst on the face. Minor lesions such as sebaceous cysts present a problem on the face when excision is needed.

Particular care is needed to enucleate these cysts meticulously, through incisions made within the relaxed skin tension lines. It may also be necessary to 'break-up' the straight incision line so that it is less obvious.

A **keloid** is a further concern, particularly in black skin. This followed excision of a sebaceous cyst in the upper neck.

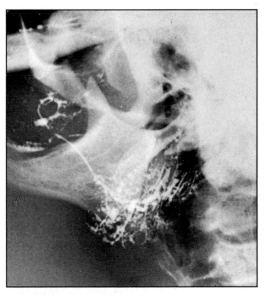

490 Sialectasis of the parotid gland. This presents as intermittent episodes of painful swelling. Calculi in the parotid duct are uncommon, and are not easily demonstrated on x-ray. An intra-oral view is necessary. A sialogram confirms sialectasis and the punctate dilations of the parotid ducts are similar in appearance to bronchiectasis. The parotid swelling with sialectasis is often infrequent and mild, and triggered by certain foods. There is no simple treatment; superficial parotidectomy is reserved for the rare, severe cases.

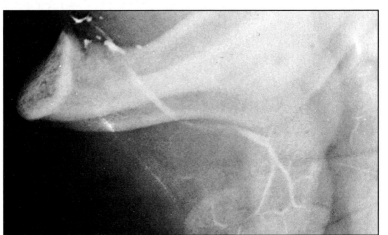

491 Normal submandibular sialogram. The pattern of ducts not involved with sialectasis is demonstrated. A parotid sialogram is not difficult to perform, since the duct orifice opposite the second upper molar tooth is obvious and can be made more apparent by massaging over the parotid gland to cause a visible flow of saliva. The submandibular duct orifice anteriorly in the floor of the mouth is not obvious; cannulation for sialography may be difficult.

SWELLING OF THE NECK

INFLAMMATORY NECK SWELLINGS

The spread of dental infection must be remembered as a possible cause of inflammatory neck swelling.

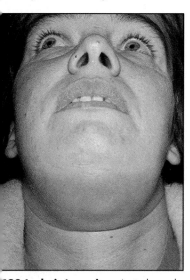

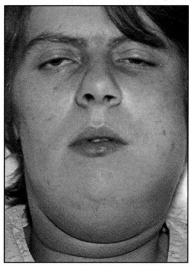

492 Ludwig's angina. An indurated, tender, mid-line inflammation is characteristic of Ludwig's angina. Bimanual palpation reveals a characteristic woody firmness of the normally soft tissues of the floor of the mouth, which is an early sign. This acute infection may spread from the apices of the lower incisors, in this case following extraction. In the pre-antibiotic era this condition was serious, because spread of infection involved the larynx and caused the acute onset of stridor. This complication is still to be remembered, although extensive neck incisions to relieve pus under pressure are rarely necessary, and the response to intramuscular penicillin is good.

493 Cervical cellulitis may develop from a dental abscess in the lower molars and involve the neck laterally.

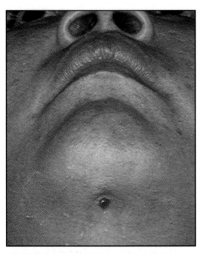

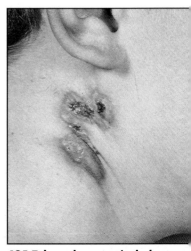

494 Submental sinus. A chronic, localised, mid-line infection under the chin is probably a submental sinus. This recurrent mass of granulation tissue formed at the opening of a sinus, leading to apical infection in a lower incisor.

495 Tuberculous cervical abscesses. These are uncommon in countries where cattle are tuberculin-tested, as intake of infected milk is the usual cause. A chronic, discharging neck abscess in the posterior triangle is characteristic of tuberculosis. Firm, non-tender nodes without sinus formation in the same site are also suggestive of tuberculosis. Che-motherapy alone usually fails to control this condition, and excision of the nodes or chronic abscesses is required.

MID-LINE NECK SWELLINGS

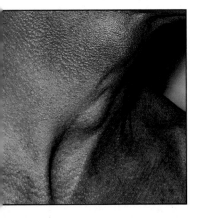

496–498 Thyroglossal cyst. This is a mid-line neck swelling forming in the remnant of the thyroglossal tract. The swelling is commonly between the thyroid and hyoid, but suprahyoid cysts also occur. The convexity of the hyoid bone and thyroid cartilage push the cyst to one side, so it may not be strictly mid-line.

The cyst moves on swallowing and on protrusion of the tongue (**497, 498**, *arrows*). It may be non-tender or present with recurrent episodes of acute swelling and tenderness.

Treatment is excision with removal of the body of the hyoid bone. Failure to excise the body of the hyoid pre-disposes to recurrence for the thyroglossal tract extends in a loop deep to the hyoid bone.

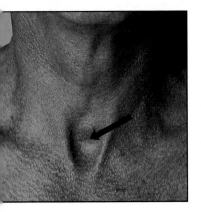

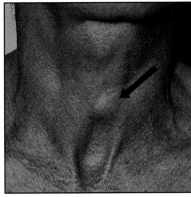

498

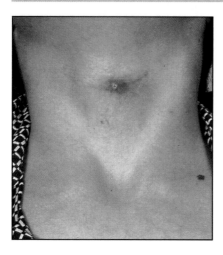

499 Thyroglossal cyst. Excision of the cyst alone, without the tract and body of the hyoid bone, leads to recurrence.

The cyst remnant causes inflammation and discharge at the scar. This appearance is characteristic of an inadequately excised thyroglossal cyst.

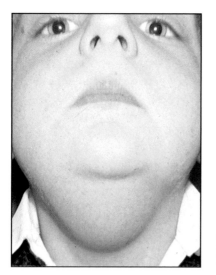 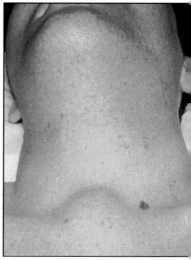

500, 501 Dermoids. Mid-line neck swellings in the submandibular region (**500**, left) or suprasternal region (**501**, right) are commonly dermoids.

LATERAL NECK SWELLINGS

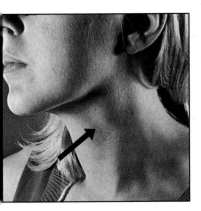

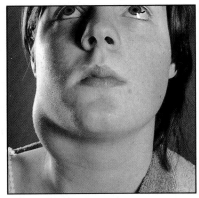

503

502–504 Branchial cyst. This has a consistent site, is smooth and, if there is no secondary infection, non-tender.

It lies between the upper one-third and lower two-thirds of the anterior border of the sternomastoid, and is deep to and partly concealed by this muscle (**504**). It can be large by the time it presents.

When excised, the deep surface is found to be closely related to the internal jugular vein. A metastatic lymph node from the thyroid, upper respiratory tract (e.g. naso-pharynx) or post-cricoid region and swellings of neurogenous origin (chemo-dectomas, neurofibromas, neuro-blasto-mas) are among the important differential diagnoses of a lateral neck swelling. The ubiquitous lipoma is also not uncommon in the neck, and in children the cystic hygroma is to be remembered. Hodgkin's disease also frequently presents with an enlarged cervical lymph node.

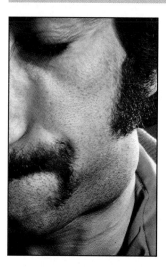

505 Laryngocele. This is an unusual neck swelling that the patient can inflate with the Valsalva manoeuvre. It is an enlargement of the laryngeal saccule into the neck between hyoid and thyroid cartilage. It tends to occur in musicians who play wind instruments or in glass blowers. Infection may develop in laryngoceles (a pyolaryngocele), and presents as an acute neck swelling often with hoarseness and stridor.

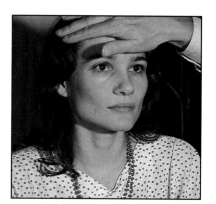 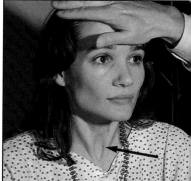

506, 507 Test for accessory (XIth) cranial nerve function. The sternomastoid muscle is supplied by the accessory nerve. If the patient is asked to press the forehead against the examiner's hand, the sternal attachments of the muscle stand out (*arrow*).

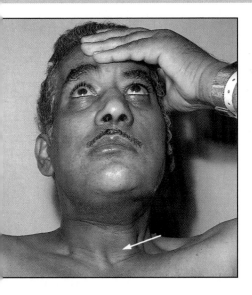

508 Test for accessory (XIth) cranial nerve function. When the XIth cranial nerve is inactive, the sternal head on the side of the lesion remains flat (*arrow*).

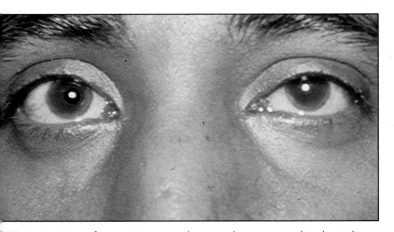

509 Horner's syndrome. Pressure on the sympathetic nerve trunk in the neck, particularly by malignant disease, causes changes in the eye. Ptosis, with a small pupil, is apparent in the patient's left eye; this is also associated with an enophthalmos and a lack of sweating. With a cervical swelling, examination should exclude Horner's syndrome.

Index